## DATE DUE

| | |
|---|---|
| FEB 2 0 1997 | MAR 2 8 1994 |
| Mar 6 , 97 | APR 2 7 1994 |
| Mar | SEP 15 1994 |
| MAR 3 1 1993 | OCT 1 8 1994 |
| | NOV 1 4 1994 |
| MAR 1993 | NOV 2 8 1994 |
| MA 1993 | |
| MAY 1993 | JAN 1995 |
| | FEB 1 1 1995 |
| SEP 2 8 1993 | FEB 2 4 1995 |
| OCT 1 4 1993 | MAR 2 2 1995 |
| OCT 2 8 1993 | APR 0 6 1995 |
| NOV 2 3 1993 | APR 2 7 1995 |
| DEC 1 2 1993 | OCT - 5 |
| | OCT 19 |
| FEB 0 9 | JAN 1 1996 |
| FEB 1 0 1994 | |
| FEB 2 1 1994 | |
| MAR 1 | |

BROD

# ANOREXIA, BULIMIA, AND COMPULSIVE OVEREATING

# ANOREXIA, BULIMIA, AND COMPULSIVE OVEREATING

## A Practical Guide for Counselors and Families

### Kathleen Zraly and David Swift, M.D.

*Foreword by William Van Ornum*

*Continuum* | *New York*

1990

The Continuum Publishing Company
370 Lexington Avenue
New York, NY 10017

Copyright © 1990 by Kathleen Zraly and David Swift, M.D.
Foreword Copyright © 1990 by William Van Ornum

Printed in the United States of America

*Library of Congress Cataloging-in-Publication Data*

Zraly, Kathleen.
  Anorexia, bulimia, and compulsive overeating : a practical guide
for counselors and families / Kathleen Zraly and David Swift ;
foreword by William Van Ornum.
      p.      cm. — (Continuum counseling series)
  Includes bibliographical references.
  ISBN: 0-8264-0490-1
  1. Eating disorders.  I. Swift, David, 1936–  .  II. Title.
III. Series.
RC552.E18Z73   1990
616.85′26—dc20                                                90-1986
                                                                  CIP

# Dedication

To Tony Papalia and the M. G. 7's.

Kathleen M. Zraly, M.A., C.E.D.T.

For my part, I dedicate this book to L. B. H. and the many eating-disordered people I have worked with during the past four years in appreciation of their trust and all they have taught me.

David Swift, M.D.

# Contents

Foreword by William Van Ornum, Ph. D.   9

Acknowledgments   13

Author's Note   15

Introduction by Kathleen Zraly   17

Introduction by David Swift, M.D.   27

1 | Phenomenology: The Tip of the Iceberg   29

2 | Personality Types: A Look Below the Surface   36

3 | Core Issues   53

4 | Theoretical Understanding of People with Eating Disorders   71

5 | The Inpatient Unit   85

6 | Drowning In A Sea Of Fear   111

7 | The Fork In the Road   120

8 | Recovery: Follow the Yellow Brick Road   130

Appendix A:  The Twelve Steps of Recovery Adapted from Alcoholics Anonymous   149

Introduction to Appendices B, C, and D   151

Appendix B: Behavioral Contract   153

Appendix C:  Information For New Patients   157

Appendix D: Inpatient Daily Schedule   161

Suggested Reading   163

# Foreword

The Continuum Counseling Series—the first of its kind for a wide audience—presents books for everyone interested in counseling, bringing to readers practical counseling handbooks that include real-life approaches from current research. The topics deal with issues that are of concern to each of us, our families, friends, acquaintances, or colleagues at work.

General readers, parents, teachers, social workers, psychologists, school counselors, nurses and doctors, pastors, and others in helping fields too numerous to mention will welcome these guidebooks that combine the best professional learnings and common sense, written by practicing counselors with expertise in their specialty.

Increased understandings of ourselves and others is a primary goal of these books—and all professionals agree that greater empathy is the quality essential to effective counseling. Each book offers practical suggestions on how to "talk with" others about the theme of the book—be this in an informal and spontaneous conversation or in a more formal counseling session.

Professional therapists will value these books also, because each volume in The Continuum Counseling Series develops its subject in a unified way, unlike many other books that may be either too technical or as edited collections of papers may come across as being disjointed. In recent years both the American Psychological Association and The American Psychiatric Association have endorsed books that build on the scientific traditions of each profession but are communicated in an interesting way to general readers. We hope that professors and students in fields such as psychology, social work, psychiatry, guidance and counseling, and other helping fields will find these books to be helpful companion readings for undergraduate and graduate courses.

From nonprofessional counselors to professional therapists, from students of psychology to interested lay readers, The Continuum Counseling Series endeavors to provide informative, interesting, and useful tools for everyone who cares about learning and dealing more effectively with these universal, human concerns.

## Anorexia, Bulimia, and Compulsive Overeating

*Anorexia, Bulimia, and Compulsive Overeating,* by Kathleen Zraly and David Swift, presents a guide to understanding and working with people who have disorders such as anorexia nervosa and bulimia nervosa. In recent years attention has focused on these problems, since many celebrities have suffered from them. There have been a number of informative autobiographies by sufferers of these eating disorders themselves. Now in one volume we have a book that defines and describes eating disorders according to the latest information available on these problems, which are common in their moderate form and, although somewhat rare in severe forms, are so destructive as to be life-threatening.

Persons who work in a counseling capacity, teachers and school administrators, others in the helping fields, and friends and family members of persons with eating disorders will find this book helpful and informative.

As a team, Zraly and Swift bring a unique perspective. Kathleen Zraly is a masters-level psychologist who experienced and overcame a severe eating disorder herself; providing the background and interest for a career devoted to helping others with this problem. David Swift has many years as a physician and psychiatrist, beginning with his training at Harvard University Medical School, and continuing through his current work at Craig House Hospital. The authors work together as part of a comprehensive team treating eating disorders, and they blend their expertise together.

Many readers may wonder, "Exactly what is an eating disorder?" The authors begin by providing and explaining the most current information from the *Diagnostic and Statistical Manual of Mental Disorders,* Third Edition—Revised (DSM-III-R). Since depression and physical problems often accompany eating disorders, the expertise of a physician is especially helpful. Some very vivid and engaging case examples portray the range of problems associated with eating disorders, and convey the human suffering and emotional cost to each victim.

Throughout the book, the authors develop one of the major themes of The Continuum Counseling Series, describing what it feels like to have an eating disorder by highlighting the underlying emotional themes and issues, as well as the various treatment approaches and programs that are available. Counselors as well as friends of eating-disorders victims will find that these descriptions help engender greater empathy and understanding.

What goes on in inpatient treatment programs, and what are issues for counselors to consider? Zraly and Swift give a detailed look at how many programs are modeled after the Twelve Step program of Alcoholics Anonymous. Family members and friends will find these passages helpful in understanding what goes on during the treatment process.

In severe cases, an individual with an eating disorder will need to be treated in an inpatient hospital setting. This book clearly depicts the many modalities of treatment that occur in the hospital. The authors describe indications for hospitalization, the behavioral approach within these programs, and the need to look for other underlying problems through talking with and counseling each person. Several innovative approaches such as the "Shopping and Food Lab" and "Playing with Food" are discussed.

In addition to the many practical features of the book, a theoretical emphasis is maintained by connecting the problems and feelings of eating-disorders sufferers with the developmental framework of Erik Erikson.

Working with those who have eating disorders is a challenging and often draining task. Is it possible to recover from an eating disorder? The authors respond, in an affirmative and hopeful manner, YES! In their clinical experience they have worked with many people who have improved or shown great strides toward recovery, and how this occurs is presented throughout the chapters of this book.

*Anorexia, Bulimia, and Compulsive Overeating* will be a practical handbook and hopeful guide for anyone who works with or knows a person suffering from an eating disorder. Kathleen Zraly and David Swift bring a great deal of experience and compassion to their work, and their insights will be helpful to everyone.

William Van Ornum, Ph.D.
Marist College
Poughkeepsie, New York

General Editor
The Continuum Counseling Series

# Acknowledgments

We wish to thank our families and friends who gave us their love and support; Barbara Wilks who spent many a lunch hour typing the manuscript; Chris Manning, CSW who shared with us her expertise in dealing with family members; the staff at Craig House Hospital for their invaluable input and feedback; William Van Ornum for not only approaching us to take on this endeavor but for always being there to answer our many questions; Dr. Jack Baker for his support and guidance; E. C. K., the Tuesday night ladies, and finally our patients whom we've come to love and respect for teaching us both what determination and motivation is all about.

# Authors' Note

Although anorexia nervosa, bulimia nervosa, and compulsive overeating occur in both men and women, over 90 percent of the people who seek treatment for an eating disorder are women. In light of that fact, and in the interest of consistency and simplicity, we have used the feminine form (she, her, etc.) throughout this book when referring to people with eating disorders. However, the reader should keep in mind that all statements made about people with eating disorders apply to both men and women and that "her" should be read as "his/her" and "she" as "he/she" etc.

The identities of the people written about in this book have been carefully disguised in accordance with professional standards of confidentiality and in keeping with their rights to privileged communication with the authors. In some descriptions, however, true facts about these persons or about their symptoms have been retained to provide authenticity or preserve the illustrative value provided by that particular case example.

# Author's Note

# Introduction

I became intrigued by the field of eating disorders only when I found myself consumed by one. My story is a typical anorexic kind—popular, well-liked girl goes off to college only to find a huge pond with more small fish than I ever thought was possible. Not having been accustomed to sharing the pond with so many others, I decided to search for a uniqueness. Somehow I never thought this search would lead to a slow but unique way to destroy myself.

When I left for college I weighed somewhere around 120 pounds and was five feet six inches tall. I never suffered from a weight problem; as a matter of fact I was the solid athletic type. My girlfriends and I would go on diets in high school, eating unsalted pretzels and drinking Diet Pepsi—and then go to Friendly's and Dunkin' Donuts the next week. Eight months later, at the end of my freshman year, I came home weighing eighty-six pounds. I'm not sure if there are words to describe how people, family, friends, and coworkers felt—shocked, scared, angry, helpless. I heard them all, and more. My attitude was, "Why is everyone so upset? I just lost a few pounds." Needless to say, this was not taken lightly. I was brought to the family doctor soon after my arrival home. I went, unwillingly, primarily to get everyone off my back. Part of my resistance, although no one else was aware of this, was because I knew what I was doing to myself; and if they were frightened by my concentration-camp look, I was even more frightened by the overpowering feeling of help-lessness inside.

I think the doctor was unnerved by my appearance. As I had predicted, he was not pleased with my health and had commented that if I were to catch a cold, my chances of surviving were not reassuring. Funny how at nineteen years old those words were meaningless. If at eighty-six pounds I perceived myself as fat, it was certainly much more difficult to believe I was in medical danger. Out of sight, out of mind. My problem was I saw what I wanted to—pockets of fat, not bone.

At some point before returning home from school I had started to experiment with eating everything I had denied myself for months, and throwing it all up. How I figured out how to do this I'm not sure. At that time, I didn't really care how, as long as it worked.

I had an "interesting" summer. The doctor allowed me to return to my summer job as a lifeguard at a small community pool. I had made the pool a summer residence since I was about age nine. My mother went and spoke to the staff letting them know I had lost "a little weight." When I reported to work the first day, the staff was, to say the least, speechless. I think people were most frightened by a sense of my fragility. I used that "fragility" to manipulate the hell out of people. When the director of the pool asked who on the staff would be interested in being the chairman of the bathing suit committee for the guards, I timidly raised my hand and within seconds it was unanimously agreed that the job was mine. I think they thought it was great that I wanted to get involved. Little did they know that my main and only motive was to be able to pick bathing suits with vertical stripes to help make me look thinner. That summer we were all in red and white vertical-striped bathing suits. I also became very good friends with the staff member who had the keys to the snack bar. I would approach Tommy saying something like, "I really feel like a Hershey bar," and before you could blink

Tommy and I would be in the snack bar loading my pockets with candy bars. Tommy would insist that I take a few extras in case I felt hungry later on. Little did Tommy know that he was helping me stock up for an incredible binge. I think he was just so excited to see me actually eat.

By the end of the summer I had gained ten pounds, only through bingeing. I had given up purging primarily because I could no longer stick my finger down my throat; I began to gag on the thought alone. I did see a psychiatrist for a few sessions during the summer. This was not looked upon as the highlight of my week, but I reluctantly appeared at my scheduled time. Unfortunately, the combination of my underlying resistance to therapy and the lack of knowledge by the psychiatrist regarding eating disorders proved to be a difficult match. Surprisingly, during the middle of a session, which from my perspective was not going well, I stated I felt as though I was wasting my time, his time and my parents' money. I say "surprisingly," because as a people-pleaser it was very out of character for me to tell someone—anyone, for that matter—how I was feeling. My biggest fear was the person would get angry and reject me.

I returned to college excited by the prospect of being able to "start over." At this point, I think I still had no clear picture of how bad I had looked when I left three months earlier, and even less knowledge of how bad (even with ten pounds added), I continued to look. I seemed to get mixed reviews from my peers. My general sense was that all were glad to see me. Honestly, I felt as though they were all perplexed by my pursuit of thinness. Almost immediately, I encountered the quiet whispers of curious onlookers. On the outside I presented this happy, everything-is-fine-now attitude; inside I was a mess. Little did anyone know that at this point I was in the worst stages of bingeing. I brought back my new "anorexic" wardrobe of size threes and fives. From bingeing during the summer I had quickly outgrown my size ones. I felt as though I was caught in a whirlwind. Half of me wished for nothing but to be "normal" and eat like everyone else; the other half felt like I was on a search and destroy mission. From the day I set foot back on campus I know in my heart I belonged at home. Home was where my support system was. The one condition regarding my return to college was that I was to see a counselor at the campus counseling service.

I began to relish the idea of talking to a therapist. At the time I was unaware what a difference a ten pound weight gain meant regarding my ability to concentrate psychologically. I made an appointment with Tony Papalia, the Director of Counseling, and began to meet weekly; weekly only lasted six weeks. Day in and day out I spent most of my time bingeing. While everyone else in the dining hall ate their meat, vegetables, and potatoes, I skipped right to the desserts. I would eat huge bowls of ice cream topped with peanut butter, granola, and butterscotch sauce. Most watched quietly, puzzled by my thinness, which certainly did not match my eating habits. Many people, primarily the females, would comment inquisitively, wondering how I could manage to eat so much junk and still stay so thin. I would have given anything to have been willing and able to scream out, "please take this junk away—it's killing me!" But a voice inside me insisted that this secret was to be kept inside. "Nobody will understand anyway, and if they do know what's really going on, you won't be able to do this anymore." So I would obediently continue to eat, knowing the depression that would follow would be emotionally paralyzing.

Approximately six weeks into the semester we, roommates and friends, went to dinner at the dining hall. As usual, I skipped over the healthy foods and hastily made my was to the dessert bar. I needed to do this with quickness for two reasons. One, I had to make sure the dessert bar was actually still there; and two, more importantly, I needed to alleviate my panic by confirming that "my foods" were actually there. I would feel disconnected and lost if I felt that I would be unable to obtain my food and even more up in arms if I thought someone else had beaten me to the good stuff. On this particular evening I binged with more intensity and determination than I had previously. The more depressed I would get, the more bingeing I would do. For whatever reason, this binge was a doozy. I returned to my room feeling nothing but disgust, anger and hatred toward myself. Each morning I would wake up saying, "Today I'm going to start taking care of myself; no more bingeing." This night had been like all the other nights for the last three months. When I returned I headed directly for the closet, something that had recently become a ritual following a binge. I would go into my closet and take out all of my pants and skirts, trying them on one by one as the tears would begin to stream down my face. Needless to say, after polishing off at least a half gallon of ice cream my stomach would become extremely distended. My "voice" took this opportunity to once again beat the hell out of me. All of my pants and skirts following my binges understandably wouldn't even zipper, much less fit. I let my friends know with a sad smile that they should go out without me. The moment I was alone a feeling of helplessness overwhelmed me and I began to seriously consider throwing in the towel. I called my parents who were three and one-half hours away and said, "Mom, Dad, I love you very much and thank you for everything, but I don't have the resources to deal with this anymore." My mother remained calm, considering her daughter was saying dying would be easier right now. We spent an hour on the phone, then she made me promise I would go find someone to talk to—"anyone," she said— "Go see if you could walk up and down a hall with the janitor if you have to." I did leave the room on a mission to find "anyone." I knew I did not want to die; I think I just needed someone to take care of me. At that point if someone wanted to put a bib on me and spoon feed me, that would have been fine. While I was searching, my mother called back only to find no one answering. Without wanting to acknowledge it, I believe deep down she thought I had done it, thrown in the towel, that is. I managed to find friends, and after explaining to them what was going on I went home with one of them. Fifteen minutes later there was a knock on the door. It was the counseling staff, my R.A., and my roommate. After much discussion I decided I would go home the next day for a long weekend to evaluate my options. That long weekend ended up actually being a year and a half. When I arrived home we had a family meeting, at which point I became honest enough with myself to own this terrible monster. With the support of my family I made the decision to stay home, eventually to seek treatment. I initially decided to not work, feeling as though I needed a break from any additional stressors. Part of me also wanted to have the freedom to binge whenever I wanted to. I ran into one big problem—my grandmother. My grandmother has lived with my parents since I was twelve. Her domain since then has been the kitchen. While you were eating breakfast, my grandmother would sit across from you asking what you would like for lunch. Then at lunch she would ask the same about dinner. It was clearly understood that the kitchen was my grandmother's. My grandmother became my single hardest obstacle. With both my mother and father working full time, I was left home with the opportunity to binge continuously throughout the day. There were mornings I would wake up knowing, by almost a tingling sensation running throughout my body, that I was going to binge. On some occasions I was able to walk into the kitchen and say, "Grandma, I really feel that today may not be a great day so if you see me going into the refrigerator to binge just tell me to get out of the kitchen." She would respond by telling me she would do whatever it took to help me. Although this approach seemed very rational at the time, within a few hours my urge to binge grew stronger and the monster became unmanageable. When these binge feelings overcame me I became a different person. I was stubborn, unwilling to listen to anyone, and downright nasty. It was at these times that I would stomp into the kitchen as though I was on a mission, without even saying a word. As I opened up the refrigerator door, my grandmother was able to sense a binge. I would have my back to her, squatting in front of the refrigerator, opening every container, and breaking off corners of everything I could get my hands on. My grandmother would watch for a moment and then timidly begin to speak, "Kathy, why don't I fix you a sandwich." I completely ignored her and became angry at her comments, feeling she was being intrusive. She would continue by saying, "You told me to kick you out of the kitchen if I saw this happening—so get up and get out." At this point, I would become enraged and slowly turn around like a monster ready to attack. I was so angry that a binge was being interrupted that I would begin to yell very nasty comments at my grandmother, who in turn would begin to cry and shake her head. The anger would be so overwhelming that I would leave the kitchen, go back to my room and slam the door. After a while the monster would go back into hiding and I would be left feeling incredibly guilty that I had upset my grandmother.

I eventually began to look for work, knowing that any unstructured time would leave time to binge. I began working for a large company, and at the same time began therapy during my lunch hours. I grew to like and trust Judy, my therapist, more with each visit. Having worked with many eating-disorders clients before, Judy was familiar with my issues as well as my tricks of the trade. We spent most of the sessions (which started out three times per week) on feelings and thoughts related to my eating and weight. Soon afterward we began focusing on other issues—mainly involving my family. Seven months into therapy, Judy sat me down, explaining we had something important to talk about. She began by saying, "I don't want to make a big deal of this, but I need to put you on a diet. You've been gaining too much weight and now need to get back to some type of normalcy." I remember vividly my heart sinking and my head spinning. I thought to myself, "She must be crazy. What does she think got me into her office to begin with?" I left that day, meal plan in hand, feeling very confused. When I returned home I shared this experience with my mother. Her face had the look of relief. I questioned this look and she stated the family had been watching me gain weight, but felt powerless to say anything to me considering the shape I'd been in only a few months back.

I continued in therapy for a few more months, addressing my struggles with eating (which at this point was probably overeating on occasion) and my issues regarding my relationships with family. I had lessened my therapy over the course of time from three times a week to two, to one, to once every other week. I remember walking into therapy on the day when it was mutually agreed that therapy was to be terminated. Walking out, I felt a strong sense of relief and an overwhelming feeling of fear about making it on my own. Therapy had been a safe place to express my feelings without the worries of being judged. Judy became one of the first people I ever remember fully trusting. I finally began to learn to trust from the inside out—something you will be reading about throughout this book.

My weight stabilized around 130 pounds. It was a long, frustrating struggle to accept that my body's set-point (that point at which the body functions on automatic pilot) had now stabilized ten pounds higher than when I first started. But, in all sincerity it was a wonderful feeling to be able to go to Friendly's, have an ice cream cone, and forget about it.

I'm not sure when I decided I wanted to specialize in eating disorders, but I remember returning to SUNY Cortland a year and a half later and switching my major from physical education to psychology. Returning to school was trying. My main goal was to accept that others would continue to question and doubt my recovery, and if I allowed that to bother me I would eventually undermine my own progress. I approached the Counseling Center staff, not for therapy, but to look for guidance and the opportunity to pursue my interests in the field of eating disorders. Initially Tony (the director) was hesitant, suggesting I allow myself more time to stabilize and get used to being back on campus. Knowing in my heart this was what I wanted to do, I continued to address the staff until finally they allowed me the opportunity to co-facilitate a group for eating disorders. This was the most rewarding experience for two reasons. First, I was finally helping others; and second, in all honesty the feelings to binge were still there, although it had been months since I acted on those feelings. I would leave group feeling the urge to binge and as I walked home I would battle with these feelings of bingeing, quickly reminding myself of all the good, healthy advice I had just given out. Toward the end of the semester, Tony asked if I would be interested in speaking to the local Rotary club about my experiences; that was in the spring of 1981. I've been speaking throughout New York State ever since.

I continued to develop a passion for the field of psychology as well as the field of eating disorders, and went on to obtain my master's in Clinical/Community Psychology following college. Since no eating disorders program existed in the Hudson Valley, I completed my master's internship with an alcohol and substance abuse inpatient unit. From there I was asked to develop an inpatient eating disorders program which has been in existence for the last four years. Thankfully, I also met and began to work on the program with David Swift, M.D., my co-author.

After treating many men and women on both an inpatient and outpatient level, we felt it not only necessary but crucial to share with you our experiences. We feel that this book will offer you a unique perspective on eating disorders. We have intentionally taken a broader perspective to let you, the reader, understand the make-up of these people. We have often discussed with each other the theory of referring to the disorders as "feeding disorders" rather than "eating disorders." Throughout the following chapters it is our hope that the difficulties revolving around the inability of the eating-disordered person to "feed" themselves self-love, comfort, and positive strokes will become far more evident than the difficulties involved in the actual act of eating.

Kathleen Zraly

# Introduction

My interest in eating disorders is relatively recent. Although I had, for many years, been especially interested in the treatment of people with personality disorders, I knew little about eating disorders prior to the spring of 1986, when I was asked to take over as Director of the newly established Eating Disorders Program at Craig House Hospital in Beacon, New York. Since that time I have learned a good deal about eating disorders, thanks in large part to my co-author Kathy Zraly and the many patients who have come to us for treatment.

This book is an attempt to share our insights and experience with others. It is our hope that what is presented here will be understandable and useful to a broad spectrum of people including therapists, health professionals and counselors, as well as people with eating disorders and those who care about them. Accordingly, we have made an effort to keep this book as simple and as free of psychiatric jargon as possible. At the same time, because eating disorders occur in individuals of diverse social class, personality type, and family background, we have tried to resist the temptation to indulge in overgeneralizations and stereotypes. The result is a kind of collage of ideas, observations, and word pictures, which we hope will help our readers gain a better understanding of eating disorders and the individuals who struggle with them.

David Swift, M.D.

# 1

# Phenomenology:
# The Tip of the Iceberg

It seems logical to begin by describing the conditions we will be discussing in the chapters that follow. In doing so, the analogy between eating disorders and an iceberg seems valid. It will be helpful for counselors, parents, and other readers to understand this metaphor in more detail. Those expert in such things tell us that over 90 percent of an iceberg lies hidden beneath the surface of the sea, leaving less than 10 percent available for easy observation. Furthermore, the submerged portion of an iceberg can vary greatly in its configuration, and the shape of the exposed portion is of little help in predicting the shape of what lies below. Eating disorders (and many other forms of emotional illness) are much the same. The symptoms and behaviors that are indicative of an eating disorder are relatively simple, straightforward and observable. Yet, as we will discuss in the chapters that follow, the underlying personality structure may vary greatly from patient to patient despite surface similarities.

The *Diagnostic and Statistical Manual of Mental Disorders,* Third Edition-Revised (DSM-III-R), published by the American Psychiatric Association, identifies three categories of eating disorders which can occur during adult life.

## Anorexia Nervosa

Anorexia nervosa is identified by the following criteria:

A. Refusal to maintain body weight over a minimal normal weight for age and height (e.g., weight loss leading to maintenance of body weight 15 percent below that expected, or failure to make expected weight gain during period of growth, leading to body weight 15 percent below that expected).

B. Intense fear of gaining weight or becoming fat, even though underweight.

C. Disturbance in the way in which one's body weight, size, or shape is experienced (e.g., the person claims to "feel fat" even when emaciated, believes that one area of the body is "too fat" even when obviously underweight).

D. In females, the absence of at least three consecutive menstrual cycles when otherwise expected to occur (primary or secondary amenorrhea). (A woman is considered to have amenorrhea if her periods occur only following hormone, e.g., estrogen administration.)

## Bulimia Nervosa

Bulimia nervosa is identified by the following criteria:

A. Recurrent episodes of binge eating (rapid consumption of a large amount of food in a discrete period of time).

B. A feeling of lack of control over eating behavior during eating binges.

C. The person regularly engages in either self-induced vomiting, use of laxatives or diuretics, strict dieting or fasting, or vigorous exercise in order to prevent weight gain.

D. A minimum average of two binge eating episodes a week for at least three months.

E. Persistent overconcern with body shape and weight.

### Eating Disorder Not Otherwise Specified

These are disorders of eating that do not meet criteria for anorexia nervosa or bulimia nervosa. The DSM-III-R cites the following as examples of this category of eating disorder:

A. A person of average weight who does not have binge eating episodes, but frequently engages in self-induced vomiting for fear of gaining weight.

B. All of the features of anorexia nervosa in a female except absence of menses.

C. All of the features of bulimia nervosa except for frequency of binge eating episodes.

Compulsive overeating is not recognized as a separate clinical condition in the DSM-III-R and is, at present, generally classified under "Eating Disorder Not Otherwise Specified." Our experience working with compulsive overeaters had led us to see compulsive overeating as a distinct form of eating disorder. Typically, these people give a history of sustained, often daily, overeating for a prolonged period of time, resulting in gross obesity. They rarely attempt to lose weight by inducing vomiting or through the use of laxatives, diuretics, or exercise. Compulsive overeaters often attempt to lose weight by fasting or dieting, but generally fail and rapidly regain any weight they do succeed in losing. Eventually their obesity significantly impairs their physical health or ability to work and

perform normal day-to-day tasks. Embarrassment and social withdrawal are common.

Anorexia nervosa occurs almost exclusively in females
and most commonly begins during adolescence or early
adulthood. In some studies the prevalence of anorexia
nervosa has been reported to be as high as one in ninety
adolescent girls. The severity and duration of this condition can vary widely. For a fortunate few, the condition
may remit spontaneously after a few weeks or months. For
most, anorexia nervosa is a chronic lifelong struggle that
often results in severe physical debilitation or death unless
adequate treatment is obtained.

Bulimia nervosa is much more common in females,
although male bulimics are being identified with increased
frequency. The female-to-male sex ratio appears to be
approximately 50:1. In various studies of high school and
college populations, the prevalence of bulimia nervosa has
ranged from 8 percent to 20 percent of the female population and has been reported as high as 1.4 percent of the
male population. Although some bulimics manage to control their symptoms and carry on fairly normal lives, for
many others the illness greatly interferes with their ability
to function.

Compulsive overeating occurs in both men and women.
It often begins during childhood or adolescence but may
develop later in life. Accurate statistics regarding the prevalence of compulsive overeating are not available but the
condition is obviously quite common in our society.

Although each of these conditions has its own distinctive
symptoms and signs, people suffering with eating disorders share much in common. Most obviously, they all suffer! Each, in her own way, is a slave to food. Each is locked
in a seemingly endless love/hate relationship with food that
often becomes the most important, most time-consuming,
and the most emotionally charged relationship in her life.
People with eating disorders are always dissatisfied with

their weight and the configuration of their bodies. They feel fat. The scales may read 80 pounds for the anorexic, 115 pounds for the bulimic, and 350 pounds for the compulsive overeater, but the numbers are irrelevant. Each is convinced that she is fat. Each feels out of control. Each judges herself to be a failure. Feelings of failure are often accompanied by pronounced embarrassment and shame and associated attempts to hide the problem from others. Social withdrawal is common. Bingeing and purging are done in secret. Loose fitting clothes are worn to hide the fat—be it real or imaginary.

Depression is a frequent accompaniment of eating disorders. Patients often experience feelings of hopelessness and worthlessness. As they repeatedly fail in their efforts to control their weight or to stop bingeing and/or purging, they become increasingly self-critical and guilt-ridden. Suicidal impulses and suicide attempts are not uncommon. Many of the patients we have treated as inpatients were hospitalized following a suicide attempt, or because of severe depression accompanied by suicidal thoughts.

Finally, people with eating disorders are all risking their physical well-being. Ten to fifteen percent of patients suffering from anorexia nervosa die as a direct result of their illness. They essentially starve themselves to death. Compulsive overeaters significantly damage themselves and shorten their life span as a result of the many well-known complications of obesity (bone and joint disease, cardiovascular disease, etc.). In bulimics, electrolyte imbalance brought about by laxative abuse, vomiting, and ingestion of substances to induce vomiting can result in death due to cardiac arrhythmias. Repeated vomiting sometimes results in rupture of the esophagus, and extreme bingeing can cause rupture of the stomach. Fortunately, these complications are rare

All of these conditions have probably been present for centuries. Anorexia nervosa was recognized as a form of emotional illness more than 100 years ago. However, it is only during the past quarter-century that eating disorders have attracted widespread interest. Outpatient and inpatient programs designed specifically to treat eating disorders have mushroomed during the past ten to fifteen years in response to a dramatic increase in the incidence of eating disorders (especially bulimia nervosa), coupled with increased public awareness and openness regarding these conditions.

There is general agreement that the increased incidence of both bulimia and anorexia is largely the result of social pressure. Since World War II our society has placed increasing value on being thin and trim. Clothing styles have steadily evolved in a corresponding manner—tighter-fitting jeans, bikini swim wear, shorter skirts, etc. Our changing ideas of health and beauty have encouraged people to lose weight by a multitude of means (diets, diet pills, health clubs, etc.). Unfortunately, an ever-increasing number of people have been encouraged to develop anorexia or bulimia as a way of conforming to social ideals and simultaneously handling (or at least trying to handle) their underlying psychological problems. At the same time, this change in society's definition of beauty and health has resulted in the compulsive overeater appearing (and feeling) more out of step with society and more isolated and uncomfortable.

Before concluding this chapter it should be noted that we do not see all obesity as being the result of compulsive overeating. Many non-psychological causes of obesity are known and others will probably be discovered in the future. Certain endocrine disorders and genetic illnesses can result in significant weight gain, and genetic inheritance is an important factor in determining each individual's "normal" body weight. Recent research indicates that people have a genetically determined "set-point" regarding weight, and that attempts to maintain weight greatly below the set-point will result in subjective discomfort, hunger, and the urge to eat. When we refer to compulsive over-eaters we are talking about those individuals whose problems with food and excess weight are primarily the result of psychological factors and not due to physical illness or genetic inheritance.

# 2

# Personality Types:
# A Look Below the Surface

Therapists, family members, and significant others who will be dealing in some way with the eating-disordered person are faced with many important questions. Who develops an eating disorder? What are these people like? What characteristics do they share in common? How do they differ from one another? Are certain types of people particularly vulnerable to the development of an eating disorder? What sort of families do they come from?

In the pages that follow we will examine in some detail the life history of three patients. We have chosen these three because they are typical of the patients admitted to our inpatient treatment program during the past three years. We hope that their case histories will give the reader a better sense of what people with eating disorders are like, and provide at least partial answers to the above questions. These cases also illustrate that eating disorders commonly occur in people who have other significant psychiatric problems and that, for many patients, the eating disorder is only one of many difficulties that must be addressed in therapy.

## Case History:
## Obsessive Compulsive Personality Organization

### Sally

Sally entered treatment at age twenty, having dropped out of college a few weeks earlier. She was living at home with her parents and two sisters—ages seventeen and six. She gave a history of intermittent binge eating going back to age seven (she recalled bingeing on leftover food from her classmates' lunch boxes during second grade), and purging through induced vomiting since age seventeen. There had been a marked increase in these symptoms during the three months prior to entering treatment and Sally acknowledged bingeing "all day long" and vomiting up to six times daily. Sally also reported progressive anxiety, obsessive fears, compulsive rituals, and social withdrawal since age seventeen. These symptoms had also become much more intense in recent months. Her obsessive-compulsive symptoms consisted of fear that intruders would enter her home and harm either herself or other family members. She attempted to allay these fears through repeatedly checking door and window locks, and making sure that certain lights were left on at night.

Although Sally had been increasingly socially isolated and withdrawn for three years prior to starting treatment, social problems were evident earlier. During grade school Sally had associated with the more studious "college-bound" kids. During high school, however, Sally spent more and more time with what she described as a "wilder group" who were less academically motivated and often identified as rebellious troublemakers. She began dating John, a member of this group during her junior year of high school and, by the time she entered treatment, rarely spent time with anyone other than John and members of her family. She described her relationship with this young man in vague and highly ambivalent terms. She characterized him as "sweet and loving" but "not really good for me," and saw herself as "too much under his control" but also as "needing him a lot right now."

Regarding her eating history, Sally recalled being unusually preoccupied with food as early as age six. At that time, if the family went out to eat, she would always arrange to be the last to order so as to assure that no one else would "get anything better than me." She recalled that her parents often became annoyed because she would study the menu "obsessively" and take a long time deciding what to order. As mentioned previously, Sally often "binged" at school on food obtained from classmates. As she grew older, Sally began overeating at home as well. Despite her preoccupation with food, Sally maintained a fairly normal weight until mid-adolescence.

Serious eating problems began for Sally around the time she began dating John. Her binges became more frequent and she began gaining weight. Often she would "make the rounds" of several fast-food establishments on her way home from school and follow that with one or two raids on the refrigerator at home. Her weight rapidly increased from 120 pounds at the beginning of her senior year to nearly 200 pounds during the summer following graduation. She began vomiting in an effort to control her weight. Her mother's initial concern soon turned to anger as food vanished in increasing quantities, traces of vomitus were detected in the bathroom, and stashes of food and discarded food wrappers were discovered in drawers and closets. To avoid her mother's anger, Sally began discarding the wrappers in a plastic bag and throwing up in the bag as well. She would then dispose of the evidence in various dumpsters around town or hide it in her car.

During the two and one-half years between Sally's graduation from high school and the beginning of therapy, she lived at home and worked at various waitressing jobs. Her weight varied between 150 and 200 pounds. She often binged and purged at work, but was able to hide her illness well and was never fired or confronted by an employer. At work, she was friendly and outgoing. People experienced Sally as "bubbly," smiling, and cheerful. She collected large tips and spent her earnings on food. At home, Sally was generally withdrawn, depressed, anxious, irritable, and often argumentative.

Sally's decision to attend college marked a turning point in her illness. Her binge-purge behavior began to escalate and she experienced increasing anxiety and obsessive-compulsive symptomatology as previously described. These symptoms had been present in mild and intermittent form since mid-adolescence, but now erupted full-blown. She began keeping herself awake at night until the rest of the family was asleep and then getting up to check and re-check locks and lights. Often she lay awake all night listening for sounds of an intruder. Although she had been self-conscious and self-critical regarding her weight and physical appearance for several years, her preoccupation with food, fat, and figure increased dramatically. She dreaded attending classes, began skipping classes during the second week of school, and stopped attending altogether by the end of the first month. She became increasingly depressed and began to consider suicide as a way out. She experienced what she referred to as "confusion" and had difficulty concentrating. She began to fear that she was "going crazy." Although Sally attempted to hide her symptoms from her parents, they eventually recognized that a serious problem existed and arranged for her to see a therapist.

Sally's family background is as follows. She was born and raised in an urban community. Her parents were middle-class and outwardly successful. They were members of a conservative Protestant denomination and Sally attended church and religious education classes regularly during childhood and early adolescence. (Sally's church attendance had practically ceased around age 17 and, at the time she entered treatment, she had not been to church in nearly two years).

Sally's father was alcoholic and her earliest memories were of loud arguments between her parents which often awakened her at night. She recalled that as a four- or five-year-old she would often sit on the stairs and listen while her parents fought. During these times she experienced strong fear for her mother's safety, as well as her own. As time passed, she experienced increasing resentment toward her father and, as she grew older, Sally would sometimes intervene to protect her mother. On several occasions she became a target of her father's anger. Despite being hit and pushed on several occasions her anger won out over her fear of injury and she intervened more frequently. By the time she entered therapy she saw her father as "a joke" and, although she resented his irrational alcoholic rages, she no longer feared him.

Sally's relationship with her mother was conflicted. She saw herself as the protector of her mother and of her younger sister as well. This role was reinforced by her mother, who often shared her unhappiness and frustrations with Sally and used her as a confidante. During childhood and adolescence, Sally felt closest to her mother during such times. Typically, Sally would sit in the kitchen while her mother cooked and poured out her unhappiness. Sally would listen and offer advice—advice which was rarely taken. These times of closeness were always followed by their opposite. When Sally least expected it, her mother would turn against her, defend her father, and, in effect, tell Sally to mind her own business. When Sally entered treatment she characterized her mother as "wanting me to listen to her problems but never wanting to hear mine" and she expressed a multitude of contradictory feelings toward her mother.

Only after many weeks of treatment was Sally able to fill in some important historical information. With much guilt and self-reproach she acknowledged that her relationship with John was a sexual one, and that she had become pregnant during her senior year of high school and subsequently given in to pressure from John to have an abortion. She had never told her parents, although her mother had "guessed" and often made sarcastic references to Sally's immorality. Sally's sexual activity and her mother's critical and judgmental response had obviously triggered the rapid worsening of her illness that occurred at age seventeen.

## Discussion

In terms of personality diagnosis Sally shows many traits characteristic of obsessive-compulsive personality disorder (OCPD). Her obsessive fears of being harmed (fears which she knew were unreasonable) and her associated rituals of checking and re-checking locks and lights are typical of OCPD. Her procrastination when ordering at a restaurant and her need to make a perfect choice and get something "better" than anyone else are also typical. During the initial phase of treatment, which took place on our inpatient unit, Sally soon revealed other obsessive-compulsive traits. For example, when asked to write down her treatment goals, Sally produced several pages of detailed writing, listing over twenty goals and breaking each goal down into a number of short-term sub-goals. When asked to prioritize her goals, she had great difficulty deciding which were the most important—as if there were a perfect order of priorities that she must find so as to feel at ease. These characteristics of preoccupation with details and indecisiveness are further evidence of an underlying obsessive-compulsive personality structure.

As Sally's treatment progressed, more obsessive-compulsive traits emerged, which were outward manifestations of her demanding superego. As is common in obsessive-compulsive patients, Sally had great difficulty letting go of judgmental anger. As a result, Sally harbored a great deal of resentment toward others (particularly her parents) and this, in turn, kept her locked in power struggles and efforts to control and change other people. At times her anger would erupt outwardly—as when she would intervene in her parents' quarrels and attack her father. For the most part, however, Sally kept her anger hidden. During the early phase of treatment she often denied angry feelings altogether, and her anger toward her mother, in particular, was so thoroughly repressed that Sally was genuinely unaware of it. Less strongly repressed and denied was the judgmental anger that Sally felt toward herself. She was locked in an internal power struggle as well—constantly trying to live up to her own perfectionistic standards and generally falling short. Guilt, self-criticism, and depression were the inevitable result.

Problems with anger and control are common in patients with eating disorders and we will have more to say about this later in the book. In Sally's case, problems with anger and control were linked to her underlying obsessive-compulsive personality structure and its attendant perfectionism and demanding behavioral standards.

### Case History: Dependent Personality Organization

#### Jean

Jean entered treatment at age twenty-eight on the recommendation of her employer. She worked as a secretary in a law office. For some time prior to starting treatment she had been having difficulty concentrating and appeared depressed and preoccupied.She had been bingeing several times a day and had gained approximately twenty pounds in the past month. Her work was slipping and she occasionally would break down and cry at work "for no reason." Jean was five feet three inches tall and weighed 185 pounds. She was a compulsive overeater.

Although Jean's parents and four older siblings were all of normal weight, Jean had been "chubby" since early childhood. At age thirteen she was five feet tall and weighed 150 pounds. At high school graduation she was five feet four inches tall and weighed approximately 200 pounds. During the ensuing 10 years, Jean's weight fluctuated between 140 pounds and 250 pounds. She had tried many diet plans and had joined a number of self-help groups. Several had been of temporary benefit. On one plan Jean lost eighty pounds in five months but then regained the weight and twenty pounds more within a year.

Jean identified loneliness as a major problem. She longed for marriage and a family, but despaired of ever achieving her goal. During those times when her weight was lowest she was often asked out on dates and had met a number of interesting and attractive men. Invariably, she eventually "lost interest" in all of them, and had either withdrawn from them or pushed them away by becoming overdemanding and critical. It seemed (and Jean eventually agreed) that being popular with men was often what triggered her regaining weight after a period of successful dieting.

Regarding her social relationships, Jean recalled that she had many neighborhood playmates and was "a tomboy" during her preadolescent years. In high school she dated occasionally, but had no serious relationships. She reported that school was "always hard for me," and she saw herself as less bright and less physically attractive than her peers. Although she got along well with everyone she had no really close friends and never experienced herself as important in relationship to her peer group. She recalled trying hard to fit in and be popular, but repeatedly feeling hurt when others failed to give her the attention and acceptance she sought. After graduating from high school, Jean worked at a series of minimum-wage jobs, continued to live with her parents, and spent a great deal of time at home listening to music and watching television. Eventually she began working as a secretary in a law office—a job obtained through an uncle who also worked there. She had held that job for six years prior to entering treatment.

Jean dated sporadically following graduation from high school. She spoke of one particular "boyfriend" whom she had been "dating" for five years and hoped eventually to marry. On closer examination, however, this relationship was more fantasy than reality. He lived some distance away and their communication was mostly by phone. They actually saw each other only three or four times a year.

Jean described her parents as quiet and stable. Both were employed at a nearby state mental hospital—father as a maintenance worker and mother as a secretary. Both were in their sixties and nearing retirement.

Whereas Jean's siblings were all living away from home and financially independent, Jean had never broken away. She had briefly lived in her own apartment some years earlier, but encountered financial problems (largely due to poor budgeting and overspending for food and unneeded luxuries), and had returned home at her mother's suggestion. She lived there rent-free, and was fearful of living on her own because of her inability to manage money and her general lack of confidence.

Jean's parents shared Jean's view of herself. Although they often said they wanted Jean to become independent they saw her as needing their continued support. They described her as different from her siblings. Each of her siblings had gone through a period of adolescent rebellion, but Jean had not. They had left home during their teens or early twenties and Jean had not. They were all married and Jean was not. They had no problems with depression or weight and Jean did. At times her parents appeared to resent Jean's dependency, but they nonetheless continued to house her and support her financially.

During the course of treatment it became apparent that Jean's recent depression and weight gain had been triggered by her parents' decision to sell their home and move out of the state when they reached retirement. Although Jean had tried to discount the importance of her parents' decision, it clearly evoked strong feelings of fear, anger, and abandonment. Unable to respond to these feelings in constructive ways, Jean had become depressed and dysfunctional and had again begun gaining weight.

## Discussion

From this brief case presentation it is obvious that Jean's personality structure is very different from Sally's. Jean shows a basically dependent personality organization. Her anxiety about living alone and her continued reliance on her parents for material and emotional support attest to her strong dependency needs. Her inability to find a good job without her uncle's assistance also fits the picture. People of dependent personality type often rely heavily on others in matters of decision-making, job-finding, and meeting basic needs for housing and financial support. Jean shows all of these characteristics.

Jean's childhood history of trying to please others and often feeling hurt and rejected by others is also a common finding among dependent people. In therapy it emerged that Jean had learned to avoid the pain of rejection by pushing others away before they could reject her. Finding fault with other people, "losing interest," and gaining weight were the techniques Jean most often employed to protect herself from the disapproval and rejection of others. At the same time, she clung to fantasy relationships which were safe. Since there was little real relationship there was little risk of being hurt.

Jean showed another trait common in people with dependent personalities. She was overly agreeable. She smiled constantly—even when describing painful events. Expressions of anger, hurt, fear, or sadness were generally accompanied by a cheerful smile. This behavior was traceable to her grade-school years and was a technique designed to please others and thereby minimize the possibility of rejection.

Finally, individuals with dependent personality disorders typically feel overwhelmed and helpless when faced with the prospect of losing an important relationship. In Jean's case, it was the news that her parents would soon be moving out-of-state that precipitated her acute decompensation and subsequent entry into therapy. So Jean, like many eating-disordered patients (especially those suffering from compulsive overeating) manifested most of the characteristics commonly associated with dependent personality organization.

## Case History: Borderline Personality Organization

### Nancy

Nancy entered treatment for chronic bulimia at age twenty-five because her bingeing and purging had escalated to the point that she could no longer function in her position as a financial aid counselor at a nearby college. She gave a ten-year history of eating disorder associated with a number of other self-damaging behaviors. Her story is as follows.

Nancy was the second of three children born to a middle-class family. Early growth and development were apparently normal. She described herself as being an underachiever who was frequently "disruptive" in grammar school in order to "draw attention to herself."

During her sophomore year of high school Nancy began smoking marijuana and often felt depressed and directionless. She experienced herself as fat and unattractive although, at 135 pounds, she was well within the normal weight range for her height. She began dieting. Her diet soon became a fast and she rapidly lost weight—to 105 pounds. The school nurse alerted Nancy's parents and she was referred to a psychiatrist, whom she saw for "a few unproductive sessions." Nancy began eating again but turned from anorexia to bulimia. She began bingeing and purging and continued to do so with varying degrees of intensity for the next ten years. Her purging behaviors included abuse of laxatives, diuretics, and amphetamines, as well as vomiting.

Despite persistent depression and her eating disorder, Nancy graduated from high school with her class and began working. She had continued to abuse marijuana during high school and now began drinking excessively and abusing "uppers and downers" as well. Three months after starting work, Nancy moved out of her parents' home to share an apartment with a female co-worker. Her drug and alcohol abuse steadily increased, and two months later she left her job and entered a residential drug rehabilitation program on the recommendation of friends. Nancy disliked the program and described it as "a stupid waste of time." She eloped from the program and drank or abused drugs on several occasions before finally being kicked out three months after she had entered it. She then lived briefly with an aunt and uncle and enrolled in an outpatient drug and alcohol program, but within a few weeks was feeling so "hopeless and disconnected" that she slashed her wrists while traveling by bus to a group therapy session. She was taken to a local emergency room by some of the group members and from there was briefly hospitalized at a state psychiatric hospital before entering a second residential rehabilitation program.

Nancy remained in this program for the next two and

one-half years. As she gradually progressed through the program she began attending college and eventually moved into a group home and matriculated as a full-time student. She maintained abstinence from drugs and alcohol throughout the two and one-half years, but continued to binge and purge episodically, and also cut herself on several occasions. Most of the cuts were superficial but a few required suturing.

During the third year of college Nancy moved from the group home to an apartment of her own and began seeing a therapist for individual psychotherapy. She attended A.A. meetings regularly at first, but soon slacked off and within three months, stopped going to meetings and discontinued therapy as well. She began drinking again and sometimes cut herself while intoxicated. During her final year of college she spent numerous evenings in the local emergency room intoxicated, bleeding, or both. She continued to binge and purge, but now limited her purging to induced vomiting. She no longer abused drugs.

Following graduation from college, Nancy's symptoms again increased. She re-entered outpatient therapy, but because of increasing depression and self-destructive behaviors, she was soon hospitalized. In the hospital she received a variety of tranquilizers and antidepressants, including lithium carbonate, Tofranil, Elavil, and Nardil. None appeared to be of significant benefit. She remained in the hospital for six months. Subsequently she returned to her parents' home, discontinued her medications, and entered outpatient treatment with a new therapist.

Bright, attractive, and well educated, Nancy had no difficulty obtaining a job in a college financial aid office. For several months thereafter Nancy did well. She was productive and well liked at work. She appeared to be using therapy well and developed a positive attitude toward her therapist. She did not drink or use drugs and her eating behaviors, while not normal, were much improved.

Then, gradually, all the old symptoms began to return—first drinking, then increasing depression and social withdrawal, followed soon by frequent bingeing and vomiting and, finally, self-cutting. The frequency of therapy sessions was increased in an attempt to deal with her worsening condition, but even three sessions per week plus frequent telephone contact with her therapist failed to halt the progression of her symptoms. Feeling desperate, hopeless, and suicidal, Nancy quit her job and entered our inpatient eating disorders program on the advice of her therapist.

To complete this outline of Nancy's history, a brief discussion of her parents is in order. Nancy described both parents as being undemonstrative and rather socially withdrawn. They rarely went out or invited guests to their home. Neither was involved in outside social or recreational activities, except that Nancy's mother participated in some local church functions. Nancy described her father as a conscientious worker and good provider, but quiet and emotionally uninvolved. She experienced him as disinterested and detached—responsive to concrete needs but "not interested in me as a person." He showed little emotion or affection toward any family members.

Nancy's mother was described as being more emotionally expressive but "passive and ineffectual," and dependent on her husband. She had worked in an office prior to marriage but not since. She never drove a car. By Nancy's description, she led a very constricted life and had no desire to change it.

During the course of Nancy's illness, her parents had become increasingly frustrated, disapproving, and withdrawn. Nancy was aware of wanting their attention and approval, but experienced them as becoming more and more detached. This perception was borne out by the fact that they refused to participate in family therapy when Nancy entered our inpatient program. They explained that they had done that before during previous hospitalizations and felt that it "did no good."

## Discussion

Anyone who has had experience working with personality-disordered patients will have no difficulty identifying Nancy as a severe borderline personality disorder. In fact, one could very legitimately say that her personality disorder is her primary diagnosis, and recommend that inpatient treatment be carried out on a borderline unit rather than an eating disorders unit. Of the three cases presented in this chapter, Nancy best illustrates a very basic truth—namely that eating disorders occur in people with significant and often chronic personality pathology, which is frequently severe enough to warrant the diagnosis of a full-blown personality disorder. (Those not familiar with personality disorders are invited to consult the *Diagnostic and Statistical Manual of Mental Disorders,* published by the American Psychiatric Association, for a concise description of these conditions).

The DSM-III-R lists eight characteristics commonly present in patients with borderline personality disorder. Nancy manifested almost all of them. Most notably, she displayed the impulsive self-damaging behavior seen in most borderlines (e.g., her bingeing, purging, drug and alcohol abuse, and self-cutting). Recurrent bouts of depression often associated with suicidal feelings and gestures, common in borderlines, were evident in Nancy's history. She also experienced frequent feelings of emptiness and boredom and a need to escape such feelings by creating excitement or drawing attention to herself. This, too, is a common phenomenon in borderlines. As noted in her case presentation, Nancy was "disruptive" and deliberately "drew attention to herself" in grade school. Later, she used food, drugs, and alcohol in her attempts to fill up the emptiness she experienced within herself. These behaviors were generally acted-out openly (e.g., school misconduct, cutting herself on a bus), and almost always drew a response from other people. (It should be noted here that Sally's behavioral symptoms of bingeing, purging, and indulging in obsessive rituals were acted-out in secret and rarely attracted the attention of others. This is a significant difference between borderline and obsessive-compulsive personality styles).

After being admitted to the inpatient unit, Nancy showed other borderline traits. She rapidly developed intense and unstable relationships with treatment staff. A staff member who was idealized one day might be the target of hostility and ridicule the next. Similar dramatic fluctuations in mood and attitude had been evident for many years. For example, Nancy had frequently entered therapy with great hope and enthusiasm only to drop out in anger a few weeks later when her unrealistic expectations were not met. Dramatic shifts of attitude from happy overidealization to hostile devaluation are seen in most borderlines and can present extremely difficult management problems for friends, family, and care-givers. We will have more to say about this later on when discussing specific treatment strategies.

Nancy demonstrated other maladaptive patterns of behavior consistent with the diagnosis of borderline personality disorder. These included intense fear of abandonment and repeated, often self-damaging, efforts to keep people from leaving (being needy, violent, or self-destructive); chronic low self-esteem and self-criticalness; and uncertainty regarding career choices and long-term goals. In short, Nancy was a severe borderline personality disorder, and had shown signs of that condition since childhood.

## Summary

Thus far we have been looking at eating disorders from the outside in. We have described anorexia nervosa, bulimia nervosa, and compulsive overeating, and have shown how these disorders are easily identified on the basis of observable surface behavior. We then looked at how, apart from their eating-disordered behaviors, these patients may vary greatly from one another in terms of their personality organization and styles of relating to other people. The three case histories presented also illustrate the fact that eating disorders often occur in people who have other significant problems which are sometimes very disabling in their own right, and are related to the individual's personality organization. In the chapter that follows we will look still deeper and discuss the core issues that virtually all eating-disordered patients share.

# 3

## Core Issues

**M**ost of our readers are probably familiar with the story of the blind men and the elephant. Each blind man was given a few minutes to feel the elephant and then asked to describe it. Naturally, the descriptions varied markedly one from another, depending on the part of the elephant each man encountered. Each described a real piece of the elephant but, after each man had shared his perceptions, the elephant remained a mystery.

Mental health professionals, as well as others who come in contact with eating-disordered people, often find themselves in the same situation as the blind men. We talk with these people, ask them questions, and listen to their stories. We spend a few hours with a person who has lived for, say, twenty years (175,200 hours) and attempt to arrive at an understanding of that person. Small wonder that the basic causes of most mental illness remain mysterious—and the subject of ongoing research and debate. With these humbling thoughts in mind, let us begin our discussion of the basic problems underlying eating disorders by looking at some pieces of the puzzle that are frequently encountered in clinical practice.

### Dependency on Parents

Eating-disordered patients are often abnormally dependent on, or emotionally involved with one or both parents.

Their relationship with parents is characterized by immature patterns of thinking, feeling, and behavior that would be considered appropriate at a younger age but, given the patient's actual age, are inappropriate. In psychiatric terminology this is referred to as an unresolved symbiosis.

In the normal course of development, the child, initially totally helpless and dependent, gradually achieves a sense of separateness, autonomy, and self-confidence. Ideally, by late adolescence or early adulthood the child experiences herself as the emotional equal of her parents. Although they may not be equal in terms of material wealth, wisdom, or achievement, the child sees herself as being a separate adult entity, free to make independent choices, having equal rights, being responsible for her behavior and its consequences, and capable of succeeding in life without parental help. Patients with eating disorders have failed to achieve these goals. They remain dependent. They continue to see their parents through the eyes of a child.

This dependency is sometimes quite obvious, as with Jean, whom we presented as an example of a dependent personality disorder. With other patients, the dependency may be less apparent. Nancy, for example, had lived away from home for most of her adult life. She was highly critical of her parents, belittled them for their alleged shortcomings, and often insisted that she wanted nothing from them. But, beneath that facade Nancy felt hurt, alone and afraid. Her dependency surfaced when her parents went away on a lengthy vacation trip while she was hospitalized. Nancy then experienced intense anxiety and feelings of abandonment, which triggered an exacerbation of her eating disorder and other acting-out behaviors, including cutting herself.

Occasionally patients succeed in establishing what appears to be a high degree of separation and independence from parents. One of our patients, a married mother of two young children, had struggled with bulimia since the age of twenty. Her relationship with her parents, while not especially close, had been cordial and outwardly conflict-free since adolescence. She entered treatment because of escalating symptoms after her father retired and her parents began devoting more time to their grandchildren. Initially, the patient insisted that she welcomed her parents' increased involvement and appreciated the attention they lavished on her children. She noted that it was "like having a free babysitter" and denied any emotional discomfort. As treatment progressed, however, this patient recognized that she deeply resented her parents for "giving my kids what they never gave me." Awareness of anger was soon followed by awareness of long-repressed loneliness and longing for parental love and acceptance. As this patient worked through these feelings in therapy, her bulimic symptoms subsided.

## Problems with Problem-Solving

Healthy problem-solving can be defined as activity which effectively ends or ameliorates an immediate difficulty; prevents or at least lessens the chance of the difficulty reoccurring; meets the real needs of all people concerned; and doesn't violate anyone's basic rights. A corollary to this definition is that when a problem concerns more than one person, all parties involved cooperate actively in the problem-solving process. Patients with eating disorders generally have not grown up in families where effective problem-solving was modeled. As a result they lack good problem-solving skills and, more importantly, they lack faith that effective problem-solving is possible. Although they may deal well with some problems, they believe, consciously or unconsciously, that other problems cannot be solved.

Many patients with eating disorders grow up in alcoholic families (Sally, for example). Such families serve as models for passivity, the enabling of repetitive destructive behavior, and a lack of respect for individual rights. In short, alcoholic family systems model problem-perpetuation rather than problem-solving. Adult children of alcoholics typically have poor self-esteem and problems with assertiveness. In their families of origin, aggression and/or passivity are the usual responses to stressful events. Their ability to trust that they or anyone else can effectively deal with difficult problems is seriously impaired.

In the preceding section we noted that patients with eating disorders almost universally have failed to resolve their symbiotic attachment to one or both parents. Consciously or unconsciously, they want something from their parents that they didn't get as children. Their childhood needs were, in some degree, not met and they are vulnerable to regression (i.e., to slipping back into child-like ways of thinking, feeling and behaving). This, in itself, is indicative of ineffective problem-solving in the patient's family of origin. The universal problem of childhood, "How can I get my needs met in this family," went unsolved. In some significant way the needs of childhood were not met, the problem was not solved, faith and trust were damaged, and problem-solving skills were not learned.

Remember Nancy? Her parents were quiet, emotionally distant, undemonstrative people. Nancy learned early in life that the only reliable way she could get their attention was to cause a crisis or be disruptive. She recalled in vivid detail how indulgent and attentive her parents were when, as a child, she severely lacerated her back falling out of a bunk bed. Her parents responded beautifully to the crisis and provided her with the best of care. Experiences of this type rapidly led Nancy to the belief that she could meet her needs for recognition and nurturing only by creating a crisis of self-injury. She continued to act out this belief over a period of many years. Nancy's "solution" to the problem was partially successful. She did get a degree of attention and recognition. But in doing so she violated her own rights and created unnecessary problems for others. Her method of problem-solving could hardly be described as healthy or effective.

## Trust and Intimacy

Establishing and sustaining close trusting relationships is often very difficult for patients with eating disorders. This appears to be the inevitable consequence of the two problems just discussed. If one's parents were unable to meet basic needs and successful problem-solving strategies were never learned, it logically follows that intimate relationships will be viewed with considerable anxiety. After all, intimate relationships present the greatest risks in terms of vulnerability and the possibility for being hurt if problems arising within the relationship are not solved.

In their work with many types of patients, therapists commonly encounter strong ambivalence toward close relationships. Many patients both want and fear intimacy, and employ a variety of defenses in their efforts to avoid intimacy and the anxiety that it evokes in them. Patients (and non-patients as well) use deliberate withholding, intellectualization, and a host of other well-known consciously and unconsciously motivated tactics to avoid the risk of being hurt, rejected, or betrayed. In addition to these defenses, patients with eating disorders have a defense not generally used by others . . . talking about food and their bodies.

If allowed to, many people with eating disorders will talk endlessly about their illness. Even patients who, like Sally, try to hide their illnesses will do this once the ice has been broken in therapy. They often describe their symptoms in a highly self-critical and helpless manner which invites the other person—friend or therapist—to offer help in the form of suggestions, advice, or other kinds of support. We will have more to say later in the book about how therapists can best respond when patients describe their symptoms at length. For now, it should be noted that story-telling of this sort generally reveals little of real importance about the patient, and is a strategy often used by patients to avoid the risks of trust and intimacy.

## Problems with Anger and Assertiveness

Many people have difficulty expressing anger in effective, constructive ways. The popularity of books and courses on assertiveness training; the rising incidence of violent crime; the well-established connection between repressed anger and various physical illnesses; even the advent of primal scream therapy bear witness to the fact that a large number of people don't handle anger well. People with eating disorders are almost all members of this group.

A number of factors may contribute to an eating-disordered person's difficulty with anger. Many come from families where their needs and feelings, especially angry feelings, were frequently discounted or ignored. Others grow up in families where angry feelings are judged as bad and as something to be ashamed of. Those from alcoholic or abusive families often report that they were verbally or physically punished for their normal childhood expressions of anger and frustration. Depending upon their innate temperament, the influence of parents and siblings, and other factors beyond their control, people raised in such families may respond by retreating and keeping their feelings to themselves, or by attacking and exaggerating their feelings in an attempt to get their needs met. In the first instance, the result is passivity, withdrawal, and the expression of anger through indirect means. In the second instance, the result is aggressive demandingness that may escalate into high-level verbal or physical confrontation.

Most of the people we have worked with do some of both. That is, they often hide their anger (even from themselves) but will occasionally blow up and express anger in exaggerated and inappropriate ways. They often express anger in indirect, self-defeating ways. They have great difficulty finding a middle ground of healthy assertiveness. The case histories presented in chapter 2 provide several examples of the non-assertive expression of anger. Nancy's self-cutting was always motivated, at least in part, by anger toward others (hospital staff, parents, etc.). The same was true of Jean's prolonged dependency on her parents. Sally expressed anger both passively (leaving evidence of purging where her mother would find it) and aggressively (physically attacking her father during parental arguments). For all three, their eating disorder in itself served as a medium for expressing angry feelings.

Eating-disordered patients need to learn assertive behaviors in order to give up their eating disorder. They need to learn how to express their needs and feelings in straightforward, appropriate ways. We will have more to say about this in later chapters dealing with the recovery process.

## The Outside-In Orientation

People with eating disorders overvalue the outside world and devalue themselves. In general, they see power and goodness as residing in other people or things and they see themselves as weak and bad. Borrowing from the vocabulary of transactional analysis, they experience themselves as not-OK and other people as OK. It is important to note that this is a general orientation which may not apply across the board. Eating-disordered patients may identify some positive attributes in themselves and are capable of seeing other people in negative terms. On balance, however, this orientation is prominent in people with eating disorders.

One obvious result of this is that food is experienced as having immense power. A compulsive overeater experiences herself as powerless to resist it. Bulimics also see themselves as having no choices. They *have* to binge and they *have* to get rid of the food through some type of purging. Anorexics attribute so much power to food that they may avoid it to the point of starving to death. For all three groups, food dominates their lives. Food has power and they don't.

The cases presented in chapter 2 provide further illustration of the outside-in orientation. Jean, for example, gave in to pressure from John and had an abortion. She overvalued his opinion and devalued her own. She discounted the importance of her own value system in favor of pleasing John and adapting to his wishes. Subsequently she experienced strong guilt and self-criticism which further reinforced her not-OK self-perception. Jean clearly saw herself as inadequate in many areas of life. She discounted her ability to support herself financially or to succeed in an intimate relationship and retreated into dependency and fantasy. Jean saw almost everyone as more capable than herself. Nancy, too, experienced herself as needy and unable to cope. She turned frantically to pills, alcohol, and a multitude of therapists and treatment facilities looking for the strength she lacked. At other times she felt overwhelmed by the demands of day-to-day life, or the victim of bad treatment at the hands of care-givers. Here again, she saw the outside world as powerful and herself as weak.

The following is an excerpt from a journal kept by one of our patients. It conveys clearly the sense of powerlessness and vulnerability this patient experienced as she struggled with her eating disorder.

I feel like a kaleidoscope sometimes. A multitude of colors which change with every hand that touches the dial. Sometimes clear and distinct when steadied by the hand. Merged and confused when the hand is taken away. If turned too quickly the kaleidoscope becomes an unreadable blur. If abused it breaks and the colors scatter in tiny fragments, never whole again.

Another manifestation of the outside-in orientation is seen in the way eating-disordered patients use food to manipulate feelings. Food is experienced as needed in order to change or avoid feelings which are unwanted or to express feelings which the individual has difficulty expressing in more direct ways. For the eating-disordered patient, food serves much the same function as does alcohol for the alcoholic. The most common example of this is the eating-disordered patient's use of food to relieve anxiety. Anorexics experience a lessening of anxiety when they abstain from food and achieve a loss of weight or a decrease in body size. Bulimics often report feeling peaceful and relaxed after bingeing and purging. Overeaters feel more relaxed after a binge.

Other uncomfortable feelings are handled in a similar manner. Borderline patients like Nancy can numb their feelings of emptiness and abandonment by indulging in their eating-disordered behavior. Others use their symptomatic behavior to allay anger, grief, or any other emotion which they see as threatening or undesirable. Food also serves as a medium for expressing feelings. Anger, in particular, can be expressed through the manipulation of food. Many bulimics leave enough "evidence" behind them to upset other people, and generally this is a deliberate (albeit sometimes unconscious) expression of anger. Sally, for example, left traces of vomitus, food wrappers, and other evidence of her illness where her mother would surely find it. In her therapy she eventually recognized that this was largely motivated by anger and a wish to strike back at her mother.

Most eating-disordered patients blame themselves for being not-OK. They see themselves as failures and often judge both past and present behavior as "bad." Their bodies are bad (wrong size, shape or weight); their eating disorder is bad (a sign of weakness and lack of self-control); past behavior is bad (too lazy, selfish, immoral, ungrateful, etc.). Self-perceptions of this sort are extremely common in eating-disordered patients, and often give rise to strong guilt feelings. This guilt and the resulting need for punishment can be acted-out through the eating disorder. Starving, bingeing, and purging can serve as a punishment for a multitude of "sins," and as a means of relieving, at least briefly, chronic feelings of guilt. (The need for self-punishment can, of course, be satisfied in many other ways. For example, Kathy Zraly in her introduction to this book describes repeatedly trying on clothing after bingeing—behavior which served in part as punishment for "bad" behavior).

We could offer many more examples of how eating-disordered patients use food to avoid, change, and express feelings. Food becomes a multi-purpose medium for people with eating disorders—a kind of panacea much like drugs or alcohol for an addict. It provides reliable temporary relief for almost any form of distress. It also serves an additional purpose which deserves mention—that of self-validation.

It seems to be universally true that all of us, no matter what we believe, want the satisfaction of "proving" that our beliefs are correct. If we believe we are right about something we want to get others to see things our way. We may believe in communism, the right-to-life movement, psychoanalysis, or that the Bears will go to the Superbowl this year. Whatever we believe, we want others to believe likewise. We want to be right. We want self-validation. The more deeply rooted our beliefs, the more important this validation becomes, and the deeply rooted beliefs that we have about ourselves are the ones we generally defend most strongly. Unfortunately, this holds true for all beliefs, even those beliefs which seem to be negative or dysfunctional. Thus, a person who deeply believes that she is a bad person will seek validation of that belief. Despite "intellectual awareness" that the belief is probably incorrect, the person who truly believes that she is bad, or weak, or not competent in some respect is strongly driven to prove to herself and, if necessary, to others that her belief is right. Some part of us feels relieved and satisfied when we succeed in doing this. In psychoanalytic terms this is defending one's ego. In theological terms it is often referred to as pride or vanity. Without a doubt, whether by genetic accident or God's plan, it is now part of human nature. Eating-disordered patients validate their basic belief that they are not-OK every time they indulge in their symptomatic behavior. The very fact that they have an eating disorder and cannot control it "proves" that there is something wrong with them. The more entrenched the basic belief the more difficult it will be for the patient to give up her eating disorder.

## The Need For Control

The need to be in control is strong in most people with eating disorders. Eating-disordered patients often report feeling "out of control" in many areas of their lives. They may see themselves as unable to control their weight, eating behaviors, feelings, impulses, social relationships, family relationships, etc. During recovery they are reluctant to make significant life changes because in doing so, they experience fear and loss of control. The word "control" comes up repeatedly in therapy sessions, and maintaining a sense of control is a matter of great urgency for most eating-disordered patients. We see this as another result of the "outside-in" orientation.

A person with a healthy sense of self-confidence trusts

that she will be able to deal with life's problems. She has received adequate nurturing, sound information, protection from excessive stress, and the needed support for dealing with age-appropriate stress. As a result, she has been able to internalize a sense of competency and experiences herself as a capable person. The healthy person believes, "I can deal with adversity; I can cope as well as other people." The person with an eating disorder, on the other hand, believes, "I'm defective; I can't cope as well as others." Since the person with an eating disorder feels weak and unable to respond effectively to problems, she strives to control her life. The key words here are "respond" and "control." People who are confident of their ability to *respond* to life feel less need to *control* life.

Consider the following example. An eating-disordered patient who is a non-smoker attended a meeting and found herself sitting among several heavy smokers. She spent the entire meeting sitting in the same chair, feeling uncomfortable and angry, and wishing the people near her would stop smoking. She was distracted by physical discomfort, angry feelings, fantasies of revenge, and indecision about what to do. She got nothing of value from the meeting and felt miserable. Later, when discussing this event, she recognized that she could have asked her neighbor to not smoke, sat somewhere else, gone out for a walk, or stood at the back of the room if necessary to avoid the smoke. Any of these options would have been healthy reponses to the external situation and to her own needs. Instead, she "controlled" her feelings, tried to control the smokers through magic (wishing they would stop), and then indulged in fantasies of controlling them by getting revenge. She talked herself out of taking effective action by overvaluing the people around her ("I'd offend or disturb them") and discounting her own needs ("I shouldn't mind this—no one else seems to mind all the smoke").

We will have more to say about the eating-disordered

patient's preoccupation with control later in the book when we focus on treatment and the process of recovery.

## Pathological Shame

So far we have identified dependency on parents, impaired problem-solving ability, impaired capacity for trust and intimacy, and several manifestations of what we have called the outside-in orientation as important issues for people with eating disorders. We will now turn our attention to what ultimately emerges as a major problem for many people with eating disorders—a problem which seems to underlie all the other problems that we have discussed. This is the problem of pathological shame.

It has been our experience that people who were subjected to a high degree of childhood trauma and who, early in life, came to believe that they were "bad" or "not-OK" in a global way have the greatest difficulty overcoming their eating disorder. Other people, whose self-esteem was less damaged, recover more rapidly (co-author Kathy Zraly for example). A few recover without treatment, given favorable circumstances. Whether recovery is rapid or gradual, an essential part of the recovery process is that the person modifies basic beliefs about herself and comes to see herself in more positive terms. To accomplish this, most patients must come to terms with a deeply embedded sense of personal shame.

The important role that shame plays in addictive illnesses has been highlighted by John Bradshaw. His most recent book, *Healing the Shame That Binds You* (Deerfield Beach, FL: Health Communications Inc., 1988), is an excellent source of information on this subject. Bradshaw defines addiction as "a pathological relationship to any mood-altering experience that has life damaging consequences." Since people with eating disorders use repetitive eating behaviors and obsessive thinking about food to alter their mood (i.e., to allay anxiety or to avoid unpleasant emotions), eating disorders clearly fall within his definition of addiction. Bradshaw is an advocate of Twelve Step treatment approaches which will be discussed in chapter 5.

In doing long-term work with eating-disordered patients, what we have repeatedly seen is that beneath their other feelings and defensive behaviors these people feel ashamed. They see themselves as undeserving. They describe their underlying nature in such terms as "horrible," "worthless" and "a monster." Labels like "bad" and "not-OK" are far too bland to convey the inner experience of these patients.

Developmental psychologists generally agree that pathological shame has its origins early in childhood development. Erik Erikson in his book, *Childhood and Society* (New York: Norton, 1968), sees the problem as beginning around age two. In Erikson's view, the two-year-old child either achieves a basic sense of autonomy or becomes burdened with what Erikson refers to as shame and doubt. Our work to date indicates that eating disorders often have their beginnings in very early childhood. Although eating problems per se do not develop until much later in life, the roots of the illness reach back to the first two to three years of life.

Not all feelings of shame are inappropriate or pathological. People are, after all, limited beings incapable of perfection and prone to make mistakes. Some sense of shame is therefore understandable and appropriate. Pathological shame is inappropriate or irrational in the sense that it is based on a misunderstanding. More specifically, pathological shame results when the child incorrectly takes responsibility for something bad happening (i.e., when she says to herself something like, "The fact that this happened means I'm bad; this is my fault"). Many kinds of early experience can contribute to a child's sense of shame. Excessive punishment, overprotection, unrealistic parental expectations, parental unresponsiveness to the child's needs, neglect, physical abuse, sexual abuse—in short, negative strokes of any kind, if too frequent or extreme, can produce the same result.

As children grow older they are increasingly capable of being objective and placing responsibility for problems where it belongs. But the very young child with her limited abilities for reality-testing depends heavily on her parents to define reality for her. In addition, because of their dependency, very young children need to see parents and other care-givers as nurturing and good, and instinctively trust that they will be. Thus, when exposed to repeated stress or traumatic circumstances, young children are especially likely to conclude that the fault lies with them. A deep sense of shame is the inevitable result.

To conclude this chapter we offer the following excerpt from the journal kept by one of our patients. Several of the core issues just presented are evident in her writing. This patient's sense of personal powerlessness over food is graphically described as is her basic belief that she is not OK relative to the people around her. Finally, her use of bingeing and purging to avoid painful thoughts and feelings is clearly stated in her concluding paragraph.

## A Day in the Life

The streets teem with activity. Business beckons. Individual people focus on their individual purpose.

I am without real purpose on this Manhattan avenue—here on a downswing of another mindless burst of loose energy. My forces have dissipated.

I feel the edge of the grey cloud of a binge. I ignore it; push it away to focus instead on the glamour of the shop windows and the glitter of the street vendors' wares. I walk; half looking for a subway, half addressing the feeling that is now nagging—tapping me on the shoulder like the haunted ghosts of memories buried alive. It's useless to fight it now.

I check the time; 10:20 a.m. I have about an hour to purge myself of the horror about to come.

The gourmet deli is before me. Muffins, croissants, and delicate pastries beckon with their cloying scent. A real "city" binge, I think crazily, comparing with the Hostess and Drakes binges of Queens.

I buy a large chocolate milk, a buttered bagel, a peanut butter cookie, and a tremendous chocolate chip muffin. I pay quickly, counting neither what I offer, nor the change. The numbness is starting.

I leave the store and tear the wrapper from whatever is on top. The bagel. I need the milk. All is geared to bringing it up later. Eating and drinking, I stop at another deli. Everything goes back in the bag as I enter the store. More mindless choices. Another bagel, a chocolate croissant, some pastries. I leave, continuing to eat, thinking of nothing else.

The people along the next few blocks see me eating. I make no eye contact. They see me eating something. I entertain the notion that they meet up with each other at some point and compare notes. I am aware of the absurdity of the thought.

One more stop before I hit the subway. A few more pastries, a couple of buttered rolls and another drink. She overcharges me but I ignore this. It's interrupting the binge.

Foremost is the absolute necessity of the impending purge. I desperately try to control the animal ravaging. Experience has taught me that what is difficult to swallow down will be worse coming up.

The feeling is now one of disconnectedness. Nothing matters but the binge. Strange thoughts filter in and out of numbing consciousness. I'm watching someone else. I remember my annoyance this morning at my father's asking me if I had had breakfast. I'm having it now, Dad, I think insanely.

Down underground, I sit on the steps and nonchalantly

unwrap more food as though just everyone sits on dirty subway steps and has a midmorning snack. I glance nervously about. A woman is looking at me. She has dark glasses, but I know her eyes are on me. I look away. I glance up; she's looking. Panicked, I move further down the platform and tear into another cookie. I cram a few more in before the train comes.

On the train, I look for the people who seem most out of it. They won't notice me.

Out comes a buttered bagel, as though I've just now gotten around to breakfast. I avoid the eyes of a blond woman who seems interested. I feel the panic again.

I'm careful with the bagel—it will be near the top and if it sticks, it *all* sticks. Each bite is mixed with milk.

I move to another seat and pretend to examine the map. I sit down and work on the biggest, dryest muffin I've ever seen. It's stale, I don't care.

The train stops and the blond woman is by the door. I freeze—wiling the panic to subside. I don't dare look up until she gets off the train. I am shaking.

My stop. My bus is not leaving. Time for a quick ice cream cone. I give him too much money. He takes his time figuring it out. The anger is here.

I slink to the back to the bus, hoping no one else will sit that far back. Someone does, and the anger deepens. I hate the man and his nearness to me. I eat the ice cream slowly. It will make it easier later.

I am sick now; really sick. My bloated body strains against my clothing. The fear is building, but I can't isolate it. I may vomit on the bus. I don't think I can handle that.

I get off the bus and stop at every deli, asking for rice pudding. I ignore their strange looks. I get the rice pudding and devour it.

I can hardly walk. I am sick and I am disgusted. The fear and the hatred are taking over. I wish I were dead.

Home. 11:30 a.m. No time to waste. I remove jewelry and clothing, dreading with all that I am what I have to do.

I position myself over the toilet, grip the bristle end of my green toothbrush and slide it slowly down my throat. Nothing. Steeling myself against the familiar panic, I probe deeper, trying to stimulate the gag reflex and praying the thing doesn't slip out of my hand and lodge in my esophagas. This is not the way I want to die.

Saliva, mucus, and streaks of blood run over my hand and down my arm. I grip the back of my leg with my free hand against the pain. My stomach finally hitches and heaves and the process has begun. Little by little, the contents of my stomach fill the toilet. The stench causes me to gag again. I continuously examine the remains with a mental checklist of what I ate and where. Greasy, stinking vomit splatters everywhere. I am glad.

I briefly wonder what I'll do if it ends up in my lungs. I have no idea.

I continue to purge, thinking of other things, wishing with my whole heart that it was over.

I begin to see and taste the first peanut butter cookie. I begin to relax. Relief flows.

I flush and carefully wash and remove all traces of vomit from the area. I disinfect with Lysol. I am careful not to get any on my hands. I cannot allow myself to think now.

Slumped against the bathtub, I rest. The tears begin to well and my throat begins to tighten. I swallow it.

One more time.

I force myself to gag again, closing my eyes against the blood. When I taste the bitter acid and the burning feeling in my throat, I stop.

I clean again, slowly, and sit for awhile on the bathroom floor. I can't think. I can't feel. I don't know what the pain is about. I check the time. 12:30.

# 4

# Theoretical Understanding of People with Eating Disorders

In the preceding chapter we examined some of the issues and difficulties that frequently emerge during the treatment of eating-disordered persons. We will now turn our attention to more theoretical considerations which provide the basis for a deeper understanding of people with eating disorders. Such an understanding should be important not only for professionals, but also for family members and others who are attempting to help and understand people with eating disorders.

There are many ways of "understanding" eating disorders. To a great extent, the theoretical orientation and background of the clinician (i.e., the clinician's belief system) will determine his or her individual preference. One can speculate at length about the symbolic meanings of bingeing, purging, and starving, and theorize as to how each of the patient's symptoms is the external manifestation of one or more intrapsychic conflicts; or one can ignore such considerations and focus entirely on changing the patient's outward eating behaviors and/or thought patterns. Most people, be they care-givers, family members, or patients, strive for some way of "understanding" the eating-disordered person's symptomatic behavior. It is difficult to measure how much such understanding contributes to the process of recovery. Some would argue that it contributes little or nothing. However, most people feel more comfortable if they have a way of explaining things in terms of cause and effect, and most therapists and patients see such explanations as promoting therapy and recovery.

It is generally agreed that anorexia nervosa and bulimia nervosa are reflective of intense ambivalence about something and that, although food is the immediate "something" in the here and now, the "real" or original object of ambivalence is something else. We see compulsive overeating as also being the outward manifestation of intense ambivalence. By ambivalence we mean that the person both likes and dislikes; wants and does not want; loves and fears someone or something. Strong contradictory attitudes therefore exist within the person, and a state of internal conflict is thereby established.

People suffering from bulimia, anorexia, and compulsive overeating express this ambivalence in somewhat different ways. The person with anorexia expresses primarily the negative or "I don't want" side of the ambivalence. Relatively speaking, her fear wins out over her hunger and the result is starvation, emaciation, and sometimes death. The person suffering from bulimia represents a middle ground. At times the positive "I want" side wins out and a binge is the result. This is usually followed by a switch to the negative side, resulting in a period of purging and/or restricting. The compulsive overeater completes the spectrum. For her, the positive or "I want" side more often wins and the result is increasing obesity. Periodically the "I don't want" side will gain the upper hand and she will restrict or diet for a time. But in the long run, her needs win out over her fears.

The question then arises as to the source of the ambivalence demonstrated by these people. If we assume that food is the symbolic representation of something else, what is that something else? Is it just one thing or is it perhaps several; and is it the same thing or things for all eating-disordered people, or something more or less unique to each individual or diagnostic group. There are no universally agreed-upon answers to any of these questions.

Eating is one of the most primitive means by which people take in something from their environment and make it a part of themselves. Usually, within the first few hours after birth, the newborn is fed, and through the processes of digestion and metabolism that which is "not self" becomes "self." The process of incorporating the outside world into the self also occurs through the physical senses of feeling, hearing, seeing, smelling, and tasting. These modes of taking in (especially feeling, seeing, and hearing) are of primary importance in the individual's psychological growth. But eating remains the most basic and essential mode of incorporation. With these observations in mind, it seems logical to conclude that eating disorders may be the end result of ambivalence about taking in something that the outside world is offering; something the individual needs and wants, but also dislikes and fears. Our view, which is shared by many others in the field, is that the feared "something" is best summed up by the words "parenting" and "intimacy," and that the original object of ambivalence is therefore the parents or other early care-givers.

From a thoretical standpoint this way of understanding the eating-disordered person's ambivalence regarding food makes sense. The chain of events, according to this theory, looks something like the diagram on page 74.

The young patient-to-be, like all of us, needs nurturing and is dependent on parents or other care-givers for survival. A close, dependent attachment (or infantile symbiosis) is established with the parent or other care-giver. Initially this may be a healthy, comfortable, mutually gratifying relationship which fosters the development of intimacy and trust in the child. But then things begin to go wrong, and contact with the parent or other care-giver is

Need For → Intimacy → Pain ⎰ → Distrust of
Nurturing     with     (physical ⎱   care-giver(s) →
            primary     or
            care-giver(s)   emotional) → Continued →
                                               Dependency
                                               and Need
                                               For
                                               Nurturing

→ Avoidance ⎱
→ and Over- ⎰   Ambivalence → Conflict
    adaptation                            and →
                                             Anxiety

→ ↑ Increasing → Symptom → ↓ Reduction
    Anxiety at      Formation      of Anxiety
    Adolescence

increasingly experienced as painful. On both theoretical and clinical grounds we know that these painful experiences or traumas begin early, often during the first year of life, and almost certainly before age four. The painful experiences may be the result of a number of factors— parental withdrawal or neglect, physical or sexual abuse, a high level of tension in the home secondary to parental conflict or alcoholism, overly critical, punitive, or demanding parental attitudes, etc. The result is that the parent or other important care-giver is increasingly experienced as a source of physical and/or emotional pain. As a result the child begins to distrust the parent, and the seeds of chronic mistrust of all close relationships are planted. Increasingly, the child experiences the parent or other care-giver as someone to be feared and avoided. This sequence of events sets the stage for the development of ambivalence.

As the intensity of the child's discomfort increases the child may initially react by becoming angry, having temper tantrums, crying, complaining, etc. But when these normal and age-appropriate behaviors fail to solve the problem, the child begins to develop defenses against the pain that all too often accompanies contact with the parenting figure. In the diagram, we have labeled these defenses as "avoidance." This avoidance may take a variety of forms depending upon the age of the child and parental response. Physical withdrawal, verbal withholding, dissociation, repression, retreat into fantasy and magical thinking, and the development of obsessions and compulsive rituals are among the most commonly employed defenses. At the same time, because the child continues to be biologically dependent and in need of parental nurturing, she learns how to get her survival needs met despite the pain that contact with the parent or other care-giver frequently entails. She learns how to please the parent. She becomes what we have labeled in our diagram as "over-adapted."

For those not familiar with the term "over-adapted," a

brief explanation is in order. Over-adapting means going along with or giving in to someone, even though one doesn't actually agree or feel comfortable doing so. Young children over-adapt out of necessity. Since a young child is incapable of moving out of the home or calling the Department of Social Services when she becomes the target of abuse or neglect, she must give in and put up with the situation in order to survive. It is a case of "If you can't beat them, join them." So the young child may learn to smile in the face of adveristy, or to be extremely hard-working and a high achiever at home and in school, or to keep her room neat and to help her mother prepare meals or care for younger siblings, or to be cute and seductive in relationships with men. But whatever form her over-adapted behavior takes, it will be motivated by her need to survive and to avoid pain, and will not be an expression of her true spontaneous self. Over-adapted behavior, therefore, begins as an act. In time it becomes a habit, a part of the individual's personality structure. By the time the over-adapted person reaches adulthood she generally has little or no awareness of the fact that she is putting on an act. She has generally repressed or dissociated most of the traumas that originally motivated her over-adapted behavior, and experiences her behavior as comfortable and genuine. As adults, people with eating disorders are very often "people pleasers." They smile a lot. They are considerate of other people's needs and feelings. They generally take the role of caretaker in important relationships. This is especially true of people suffering from compulsive overeating and bulimia, but is a prominent personality trait in many anorexics as well.

As we have indicated in the diagram, the contradictory attitudes of attraction and avoidance experienced in relationship to the parent or other care-giver form the basis of the ambivalence that is so evident in people with eating disorders. If the child's avoidant and over-adapted behaviors worked perfectly, all would be well and there would be no further problems. Unfortunately, this is never the case. Since over-adapted behavior is an act and not an expression of the person's true self, it is never completely satisfying. Also, the various avoidant behaviors previously discussed serve to minimize pain, but never eliminate it. As a result, a continued state of conflict and anxiety persists.

Most eating-disordered people begin showing symptoms of their eating disorder during adolescence or early adulthood. Although some problems with eating and/or weight may be evident earlier, full-blown symptoms usually appear after the onset of puberty. It has long been postulated that the pressures to grow up, separate from parents, establish intimate relationships outside of the family, and eventually become self-supporting are what trigger the development of clinical illness. It is easy to see why this would be the case. Children destined to develop an eating disorder approach adolescence ill-prepared to negotiate the developmental steps that lie ahead. They have not yet mastered many of the tasks of earlier developmental stages. Their capacity for trust is impaired because their parents have not provided adequate parenting. Their capacity for intimacy is impaired because they associate intimacy with pain and anxiety. They have a poor sense of their own identity because they have had to repress and dissociate large portions of their experience, and because they have largely gotten along by pretending and over-adapting. Their true self has not been allowed to develop. They truly do not know who they are, although they may pretend to know and may often believe that they do. As we discussed earlier in chapter 3, they feel defective, bad, and ashamed. As adolescence and adulthood approach, their anxiety increases. On some level they recognize that they are not prepared to go on; that they cannot meet the demands of adult life.

It might be useful to some of our readers to pause at this point and briefly review the stages of normal child development. There are several ways of conceptualizing these developmental stages. We have found the ideas developed by Erik Erikson to be particularly useful in understanding people with eating disorders. The following table is taken from Erikson's book, *Childhood and Society,* which was referred to earlier.

**Infant**

| *Trust* | *Versus* | *Mistrust* |
|---|---|---|
| Ease in feeding | | Withdrawal into |
| Depth of sleep | | schizoid and |
| Relaxation of bowels | | depressive states |
| The first social achievement allows mother out of sight without undue anxiety or rage | | |

**Toddler**

| *Autonomy* | *Versus* | *Shame and Doubt* |
|---|---|---|
| Self-control without loss of self-esteem | | Low self-esteem |
| Good will and pride | | Secretiveness |
| Rightful dignity | | Feelings of |
| Lawful independence | | persecution |
| Sense of justice | | |

**Preschooler**

| *Initiative* | *Versus* | *Guilt* |
|---|---|---|
| Loving | | Hysterical denial |
| Relaxed | | Paralysis, inhibition, |
| Bright in judgment | | or impotence |
| Energetic | | Overcompensatory |
| Task-oriented | | showing off |
| | | Psychosomatic disease |
| | | Self-righteousness |
| | | Moralistic surveillance |

**School-aged**

| *Industry* | *Versus* | *Inferiority* |
|---|---|---|
| Productivity | | Sense of inadequacy |
| Task completion | | Mediocrity |
| Steady attention | | Self-restriction |
| Perseverance | | Constricted horizons |
| Manipulation of tools | | Conformity |

**Adolescent**

| *Identity* | *Versus* | *Role Confusion* |
|---|---|---|
| Idealistic | | Delinquency |
| Integration of identification with libidinal vissicitudes | | Psychotic episodes |
| | | Doubt and sexual identity |
| Integration of aptitudes with opportunity | | Overidentification with heroes, cliques, and crowds |
| Confidence | | |

**Young Adult**

| *Intimacy* | *Versus* | *Isolation* |
|---|---|---|
| Commitment | | Self-absorption |
| Sacrifice | | Distancing behaviors |
| Compromise | | Character problems |
| True genitality | | |
| Work productivity | | |
| Satisfactory sex relations | | |

Table based on Epigenetic Chart from *Childhood and Society,* Second Edition, by Erik H. Erikson, by permission of W. W. Norton & Company, Inc. Copyright 1950, © 1963 by W. W. Norton & Company, Inc. Copyright renewed 1978 by Erik H. Erikson.

In the table, the left-hand column shows the normal or desired accomplishment for each developmental stage and its behavioral manifestations. During infancy, for example, the healthy child will develop a capacity for trust which will be manifested by easy feeding, sound sleeping, relaxed bowel habits, and the ability to tolerate mother's absence without becoming upset. The right-hand column lists the usual results of the child's failure to accomplish the normal developmental task for each stage. For infancy, failure to develop a capacity for trust results in mistrust, which is often manifested by withdrawal and depression.

It should be kept in mind that the table is not to be interpreted rigidly. The capacity for trust, for example, is not fully developed during infancy and thereafter invulnerable to attack. What the table indicates is that the capacity for trust normally *begins* to develop during infancy and that developing the capacity for trust is the most important psychological task during the infancy period. Significant traumas and betrayals during later developmental stages may result in a damaged capacity for trust even if all goes well during the infancy period.

From Erikson's formulations it is easy to see why the tasks of adolescence and young adulthood are so difficult and anxiety-provoking for people destined to develop eating disorders. Although these people often receive adequate parenting during infancy, they frequently begin to experience significant difficulty during the toddler and preschool years. Thus they often approach adolescence burdened by difficulty in trusting, a strong sense of shame, and an exaggerated sense of personal failure, guilt, and inadequacy. The challenge of establishing a solid sense of personal identity and healthy intimate relationships often seems overwhelming and the result is increasing anxiety. It is this mounting anxiety that serves as the stimulus for symptom formation.

One of the most important functions of behavioral symptoms is the reduction of anxiety. Phobias, compulsive rituals, obsessive thought patterns, addictions, and other repetitive abnormal or "symptomatic" behaviors serve to lessen the individual's level of anxiety. Although a symptom may, in and of itself, cause serious problems and significantly limit the individual's ability to function, one result of symptom formation is always to help the individual feel better. Were this not so; if behaving "normally" were more comfortable than being symptomatic, few people would ever become ill. Such problems as addictions, phobias, many forms of depression, and a host of other psychological illnesses would simply not exist. Organic illnesses and conditions primarily caused by genetic inheritance would still occur, but many illnesses, including eating disorders, would disappear.

People develop eating disorders, therefore, as a way of lessening anxiety. Although the person suffering from an eating disorder may be very uncomfortable and highly motivated to recover from her illness, it can be safely assumed that she feels less anxious with her illness than without it, and that any attempt to make her give up her illness will meet with significant resistance. The extreme life disruption that eating disorders often cause, and the high level of emotional discomfort that people with eating disorders experience as a result of their illness give us some sense of the level of anxiety that underlies their illness.

It has often been postulated that a major source of anxiety for people with eating disorders is the pressure to establish a mature sexual identity and to have intimate relationships with people outside the family. As Erikson's table indicates, these are important developmental tasks for the adolescent and young adult person in our society. Since Erikson's formulations were published over twenty years ago, the sexual revolution which began after World War II has continued and the social pressures to "grow up" and become sexually active have greatly increased. It is tempting to postulate that people develop eating disorders as a way of avoiding sexuality; that they have a primary and intimate relationship with food rather than face the anxiety associated with close interpersonal relationships; and that their ambivalence about sexuality is displaced onto food. Since they feel incapable of controlling sexual relationships, they substitute food for people and try to control food. While this theory does fit for some eating-disordered people, we find it rather simplistic and superficial. As we see it, the roots of most eating disorders go back to earlier developmental stages where trust and autonomy were the crucial issues. Pressures to become sexually mature and active may serve to trigger the illness, but are not the basic cause of eating disorders.

A bit more should be said about the final step in our diagram, i.e. "reduction of anxiety." Eating disorders serve to reduce anxiety in several ways. We have already noted that eating disorders provide a relatively safe, comfortable, and controllable object which substitutes for people, who are seen as unsafe and uncontrollable. Another mechanism by which anxiety is reduced is through regression. People with bulimia and compulsive overeating sometimes report that when they are bingeing they are "in another world" and have little awareness of what is going on around them. Their focus is entirely on food. All other concerns disappear and they seem to be, as one patient put it, "in a trance." Several patients refer to the subjective experience of bingeing as being "in la-la land." They feel much like what we presume a nursing infant feels; relaxed, oblivious to surroundings, focused on the act of eating and the comfort that it brings. Thus the act of bingeing fosters regression to an earlier infantile stage of developmental where the individual experienced comfort, safety, and trust.

Eating disorders also reduce anxiety by providing the person with an excuse for avoiding things. As one patient put it, "If I have binged or purged I can turn down social invitations without feeling guilty." She referred to her bulimic symptoms as her "cop-out," and recognized that her illness brought her relief from guilt. Finally, during their therapy, many eating-disordered persons become aware of how they use their illness in interpersonal situations. Like any illness, eating disorders can be used to control other people and to express anger or get revenge. Demands for attention and hostile impulses which the individual cannot express directly can be expressed through the illness itself, with resulting lessening of tension and anxiety. Thus a number of "secondary gains" are possible and, to the extent that such gains are present, the illness becomes more entrenched.

In going through this chapter, the reader might get the impression that all eating disorders are symptomatic of serious early childhood traumas and that the parents of people with eating disorders were all guilty of gross negligence or abuse. This is not always the case. There are all degrees of eating disorder ranging from mild transient disturbances to chronic lifelong illnesses. As we noted earlier, some people recover spontaneously and others respond well to relatively brief outpatient treatment. While we believe that most eating-disordered people have experienced some significant difficulties during the first few years of life, their childhood traumas were not necessarily extreme or unusual. There is much we don't understand about emotional illness. Individual sensitivity to traumatic events apparently varies greatly among children but we have, as yet, no accurate way of predicting or measuring such sensitivities.

We do know that some people experience what appears to be extreme childhood trauma without developing serious emotional illness, and that others, whose childhoods appear to have been much better, fall victim to eating disorders or other forms of emotional illness. The most crucial variable in determining whether or not a traumatic event will cause lasting damage seems to be the availability of emotional support. Children can cope with what, on the surface, appear to be highly traumatic events provided they have a parent or other significant care-giver who is understanding, accepting of the child's feelings, and able to offer protection and an age-appropriate explanation of the event.

Studies of people who experience extreme childhood trauma (rape, witnessing wartime atrocities, death of loved ones, etc.) show that those children who had a trusted, capable care-giver available to them were able to come through the trauma relatively unscathed. Conversely, less fortunate children subjected to similar stress often show evidence of serious psychological damage later in life. Thus, the child's ability to trust and the availability of supportive care-givers seems to be more important than the nature of the trauma itself.

For children destined to develop eating disorders, adequate support is often not available. Even when support is available, these children have difficulty reaching out for it because of their impaired capacity for trust and their strong sense of personal shame and unworthiness.

# 5

# The Inpatient Unit

In response to the recent dramatic increase in the incidence of eating disorders, many psychiatric hospitals have developed separate programs and, in some cases, physically separate units for eating-disordered patients. Several rather distinct treatment approaches are currently being used in these programs. At other hospitals, eating-disordered patients are mixed in with other psychiatric patients and receive less individualized or specialized treatment. There are, therefore, many variations and combinations of treatment available. In this chapter, we will present a brief overview of some of these approaches and then describe in more detail the program we have developed over the past four years. We hope that this knowledge can allay the anxiety of counselors, family members, and the person with the eating disorder herself, when faced with the need to enter an inpatient program.

## Twelve Step Programs

Since its humble beginnings in the 1930s, Alcoholics, Anonymous has grown into a worldwide fellowship that has served millions of alcoholics. In more recent years Alcoholics Anonymous has reached out to people with other problems as well (e.g., Narcotics Anonymous, Gamblers Anonymous, and Overeaters Anonymous).

Treatment programs utilizing the Twelve Steps and Twelve Traditions of Alcoholics Anonymous have become the mainstay of most residential and inpatient programs treating alcohol and substance abuse. This approach is now being used as the basis for some inpatient eating disorder programs as well. Many compulsive overeaters, bulimics, and anorexics have derived lasting benefit from such programs. In the past, some mental health professionals and patients argued that the A.A. approach was not appropriate for people with eating disorders, since total abstinence, which is the basic goal for alcoholics, addicts, and compulsive gamblers, could not be a goal for people with eating disorders. However, the good results of such programs demonstrates that the Twelve Step approach is useful for these patients.

Twelve Step programs appear to work because they deal directly with the eating-disordered person's underlying sense of personal badness. Twelve Step programs emphasize group interactions over individual and/or family treatment models, and each patient is repeatedly validated and supported by other group members. Their "I'm not-OK" beliefs are directly confronted and corrected by both group leaders and co-patients and the development of healthy self-esteem is consistently reinforced. In addition, the emphasis on spiritual values and belief in a higher power provides a powerful antidote for the eating-disordered person's self-shaming beliefs. The belief that one is the creation of a caring God is clearly incompatible with the belief that one is basically flawed and worthless.

Control issues are also directly addressed in Twelve Step programs. As we noted earlier, people with eating disorders put inordinate effort into trying to control their lives. They see themselves as flawed, unable to respond well to stress, and therefore as needing to eliminate stress by controlling the circumstances of their lives. This "need" to control also derives from the belief that they must hide their flaws from other people in order to avoid criticism and rejection. Their reasoning goes something like this: "I'm a bad, inadequate person who can't cope with life as well as other people. Therefore I must do two things. I must control the outside world so my life will run smoothly, and I must control my behavior so others won't see my flaws and dislike me." Twelve Step programs directly confront these dysfunctional beliefs by encouraging people to acknowledge and accept their powerlessness; give up attempts at perfectionistic control ("let go and let God"); and turn their will and their lives over to a higher power.

For those not already familiar with A.A., O.A., and related programs, the Twelve Steps common to these programs are listed in Appendix A. Suffice it to say that Twelve Step programs based on the A.A. model are proving to be a valuable basis for the treatment of eating disorders.

## Behavioral Approaches

There is general agreement among mental health professionals that useful psychotherapy cannot take place while a patient continues to indulge in symptomatic behaviors. If the patient continues to avoid or discharge uncomfortable feelings by acting-out, she will have little motivation to become involved in the difficult process of self-examination, heightened awareness of painful traumas and conflicts, and the assumption of responsibility for conflict resolution and personal change that psychotherapy entails. Since the advent of modern psychiatry during the nineteenth century, psychotherapists have been concerned with the problem of how to get the patient to "stop acting and start feeling."

Modern behavioral therapy places heavy (and sometimes virtually total) emphasis on changing the patient's "observable and measurable" behavior. Insight-oriented or "uncovering" psychotherapy is seen as being of less importance than behavioral change. In its more extreme forms, behavioral therapy concerns itself only with achieving such external change. Some behavioral therapists ignore or even discourage any attempts on the patient's part to explore past events and understand themselves in terms of their life history. The assumption is that if one can significantly change behavior, the patient's thoughts, feelings, attitudes, and beliefs will follow along automatically in due time.

Inpatient eating disorder programs vary considerably one from another as regards the emphasis placed on controlling the patient's behavior. In some programs, patients are allowed to binge, purge, starve, etc. within wide limits, provided that there is no immediate risk to their physical health. At the other extreme are programs which place very strict controls on eating behaviors by utilizing nasogastric tube feeding to ensure proper caloric intake and constant nursing observation to ensure that the patient does not purge. In more behaviorally oriented programs, hospital privileges such as permission to use a telephone, see visitors, or participate in recreation activities are contingent on the patient's eating behaviors and/or weight change. In such a program, for example, an underweight anorexic patient might be allowed telephone privileges after gaining five pounds, and visiting privileges after gaining an additional five pounds. Eventually such a patient could "earn" the privilege of participating in an aerobic exercise class and, later on, the privilege of spending a few hours out of the hospital with family or friends. Conversely, a loss of weight would result in a loss of one or more privileges.

In programs of this type, specific "behavioral contracts" are drawn up for each patient which spell out in detail what the patient must do to progress through the program and what the consequences of unhealthy behavior will be. Depending on the nature of the patient's symptoms, other behaviors unrelated to eating may be addressed in the behavioral contract (e.g., compliance with hospital guidelines, self-injury, inappropriate social behavior, etc.). A thorough behavioral contract which addresses all of the patient's symptomatic behaviors can be a rather lengthy and involved document. This is especially true for patients like Nancy, the borderline patient presented in chapter 2. In her case, a behavioral contract could address such behaviors as bingeing, purging, self-cutting, inappropriate attention-seeking social behavior, alcohol abuse, and unacceptable verbal and physical expressions of anger. For each of these categories the contract would describe the acceptable or desired behavior, the "rewards" to be given for behaving in the desired manner, and the consequences that would result from unacceptable behavior. A possible behavioral contract for Nancy can be found in Appendix B.

Ideally, behavioral contracts are negotiated and the patient is a cooperative and willing participant in its creation. Sometimes, with highly resistant patients, the contract must be imposed on the patient by treatment staff. The final results are probably equally good either way, provided that the contract is reasonable and the treatment staff demonstrate genuine respect and caring for the patient.

We see behavioral contracts as useful and necessary for some hospitalized patients. In point of fact, whenever a person is admitted to any psychiatric hospital for any reason, certain restrictions automatically apply. Hospital and unit policies, designed to ensure the health and safety of staff and patients, are imposed on one and all. But beyond those rules and guidelines that apply to all patients, specific contracts which address the symptoms of individual patients are sometimes indicated. In our work with hospitalized patients we have used behavioral contracts (or, as we call them, "contingency contracts") to address those behaviors which we believe the patient must modify before meaningful psychotherapy can take place. We see behavioral contracts, especially those that are imposed upon the patient rather than negotiated, as reinforcing the "outside-in orientation" that people with eating disorders bring to their therapy. Also; with some patients such as Sally, behavioral contracting may reinforce obsessive-compulsive tendencies which are already a significant problem. Despite these reservations, there are certainly times when behavioral contracts are useful and perhaps even necessary. We will have more to say about our use of behavioral contracts later on.

## Medication

In recent years, antidepressants have been used quite frequently in treating eating disorders. The rationale for prescribing antidepressants is two-fold. First, many people suffering from eating disorders are depressed to a significant degree. Feelings of hopelessness, inadequacy, and failure are frequently reported. Social withdrawal, lack of energy, and sleep disturbances are not uncommon. The history of suicidal thoughts is fairly common and suicide attempts are sometimes the precipitating event leading to hospitalization. In our own experience, significant depression as measured by both psychological testing and clinical evaluation has been present in over ninety percent of people hospitalized for an eating disorder. A second rationale for prescribing antidepressants is that, according to some investigators, there is a higher-than-normal incidence of affective disorders in the parents and grandparents of people with eating disorders. Since it is believed that some forms of affective disorders are inherited, it is theorized that eating disorders and affective disorders may be genetically linked and that antidepressants may, therefore, be useful even in the absence of clinical depression.

In clinical trials, antidepressants have been prescribed

for fairly large numbers of people suffering from anorexia and bulimia. The findings to date indicate that people with bulimia often respond well. Improvement has been reported in bulimic patients who are not clinically depressed as well as in those with significant depression. Anorexic patients respond less well to antidepressants. The usefulness of antidepressants in treating compulsive overeaters has not yet been systematically studied.

Many articles have appeared recently in both professional journals and the lay press about a new antidepressant called Prozac. Although it has only been available for two years, Prozac is now the most widely prescribed antidepressant in the United States. Because it is new, no long-term studies have yet been conducted, but Prozac appears to be of benefit to many people with eating disorders. Since Prozac causes fewer side-effects than other antidepressants it is generally well tolerated and is now the drug most frequently prescribed for eating disorders.

In-patient programs vary in their reliance on antidepressants. Short-term programs tend to place more emphasis on the use of these drugs. Our experience has been that antidepressants appear to be of benefit to some people suffering from bulimia and compulsive overeating. Those patients who are the most depressed seem to respond best. It is often difficult to separate the effect of medication from the effect of the other therapies that the person is receiving. Our overall impression is that medication can be of benefit, but that psychotherapy is necessary to bring about lasting change and full recovery.

## Psychotherapeutic Approaches

Traditional "insight-oriented" or "uncovering" psychotherapy seeks to make the patient more aware of the chain of life experiences that has resulted in the development of their eating disorder. The eating-disordered person is encouraged to recognize the purpose of her disorder; how it protects her; what feelings she expresses through her symptoms; how her symptoms reduce anxiety, etc. Childhood events that shaped the individual's basic beliefs about herself and the world around her are explored and related in a cause-and-effect way to the present illness. As an important part of this uncovering process, the person is encouraged to experience and express feelings which had previously been repressed, disowned, or avoided. The dysfunctional and self-defeating aspects of the individual's beliefs and behaviors are examined and healthy alternatives are identified. Broadly stated, the goal of psychotherapy is honest and more complete awareness of self and others in both the past and the present. The rationale for such therapy is that knowledge is power; that deeper and more accurate understanding makes problem solving easier; that it is easier to fix something if you know what's broken.

Inpatient programs place varying emphasis on insight-oriented therapy with eating-disordered patients. During the past few years the cost of hospital care has increased dramatically and many insurance plans (both public and private) have cut back on benefits and placed more restrictive limits on psychiatric care in particular. Insurance company criteria for hospital admission and for continued hospital stays have been made increasingly difficult to meet. As a result, lengthy hospital stays are financially impossible for many people and the average length of stay in both public and private psychiatric hospitals has dropped dramatically.

Probably as a consequence of the pressure to minimize hospital stays, many hospital programs have been placing more emphasis on behavioral therapies and medication because these approaches often bring about more rapid change in the presenting symptoms. More traditional psychotherapeutic approaches, which usually are slower to produce behavioral change, remain the mainstay of most outpatient treatment.

## Our Inpatient Program

Our inpatient Eating Disorders Program was started in 1985 and has undergone several modifications since that time. The description that follows reflects the program as it currently exists. Further changes will probably be made in the future as we continue to search for better ways of helping people overcome serious eating disorders.

### *Criteria For Admission*

There are basically two reasons for choosing inpatient treatment rather than outpatient treatment. The first is because it would be dangerous for the person to remain out of the hospital; the second is because the person is unable to carry out her normal responsibilities and day-to-day activities even with the support of outpatient treatment. Often, both criteria are present at the time of hospitalization. More specifically, some of the most commonly encountered indications for hospitalization are as follows:

1. Weight loss of twenty-five percent or more of normal body weight.
2. A longstanding (six months or more) pattern of starving, bingeing and purging, or compulsive overeating.
3. The individual cannot carry on normal activities and responsibilities because of their eating disorder (parenting, school, social activities, job, etc.).
4. Severe family conflict and family disintegration resulting from the individual's eating disorder.
5. Extreme hopelessness and helplessness.
6. Suicidal risk (impulses, plans, attempts, threats, etc.).

7. Physical complications (gastrointestinal bleeding, weakness, physical problems secondary to obesity, laxative dependency, etc.).
8. Metabolic complications (electrolyte imbalance, dehydration, impaired kidney function, etc.).
9. Failure of outpatient treatment to bring about improvement in any of the above within a reasonable length of time.

The degree of risk and urgency of any individual's situation will depend, in part, upon their living situation, their social support system, the availability of outpatient treatment, their medical history, and a number of other variables. For example, a college student who has to drop out of school because of bulimia nervosa might do well without hospital treatment, provided that her family is supportive and that outpatient treatment is available. Another student with similar symptoms might require hospitalization because of a lack of social and/or medical support. The decision to admit or not admit is sometimes a difficult one because of the many relevant factors that come into play.

### Length of Stay

The average length of stay in our inpatient program is approximately two months. Our experience has been that hospital stays of less than three weeks rarely result in significant improvement and we urge people coming into our program to plan on staying for at least one month. By four to five weeks, most of the people we have worked with show some improvement and have learned enough about themselves and their illness so that they could function better outside the hospital than they were functioning prior to admission. By six to eight weeks a majority of patients are ready for discharge. That is, they have improved to the point that they no longer meet any of the criteria for admission and their chances of continuing their recovery with the support of outpatient treatment are reasonably good. Our experience has been that people who leave the hospital earlier than six weeks have a much more difficult time and a higher incidence of relapse than those who stay longer than six weeks. These are only rough rules of thumb and a given individual may not fit the rule.

We have worked with several patients who required two or three admissions to our program before they were able to continue their recovery on an outpatient basis. Sally, for example, was hospitalized three times for a total of eleven months during a two-year period. Following each hospitalization she did fairly well for awhile and then relapsed. She used the hospital well, however, and each admission was shorter than the one before. Each time she was able to gain new ground and develop new coping skills. She has now been out of the hospital for well over a year, is working, and is continuing her recovery in outpatient treatment.

### The Initial Evaluation

Whenever possible, people interested in entering our eating disorders program are scheduled for a pre-admission meeting with members of the treatment team. The prospective patient is encouraged to bring her parents, spouse, or other "significant others" to the meeting as well. Members of the treatment team attending the meeting generally include the program coordinator, psychiatrist, social worker, and a nurse—so the gathering is sometimes quite large. The meeting is relatively informal. Basic information about the prospective patient is gathered and the structure of the program is explained. The team members describe their roles and answer questions. The prospective patient and family members are given a tour of the hospital facilities. Some beginning work is done on identifying problems and setting realistic treatment goals. This meeting establishes the foundation for the therapeutic work that will follow. By including family members we attempt to reinforce the importance of family involvement in the treatment process, and to encourage more open communication between the eating-disordered person and the important people in her life.

At the pre-admission meeting the prospective patient is given written information about the program. This "Information for Patients" provides a brief description of the program and addresses issues of concern to the prospective patient and family members. A copy of the "Information for New Patients" can be found in Appendix C.

All people coming into our inpatient program are admitted to the hospital's closed unit. This is a twenty bed unit with a relatively large number of nursing personnel, which allows for a great deal of individual attention and support. While on this unit patients are closely monitored. After an initial settling-in period (generally one to three days), people in the Eating Disorders Program are allowed off the unit to attend group therapy sessions and other therapeutic activities. However, they are escorted to and from off-unit activities by a staff member to ensure against unauthorized visits to bathrooms or to areas in the hospital where food is available. Later, when an individual has demonstrated sufficient control over impulses to binge, purge, or act-out in other self-injurious ways, she will be moved to the hospital's open unit and will be allowed to come and go within the hospital without an escort.

The initial evaluation, which begins with the pre-admission interview, is completed while the individual is living on the closed unit. The basic components of the initial evaluation are listed in Appendix C. Physical examination, laboratory tests, psychological testing, and the observation of the nursing staff and members of the treatment team are all important sources of information. Weekly treatment team meetings provide opportunity for information-sharing and planning treatment. Although the initial evaluation is generally completed within two weeks of admission, the evaluation process continues throughout the patient's hospital stay, and treatment plans are constantly reviewed and revised by the treatment team.

We mentioned earlier that the process of problem identification and goal-setting begins during the pre-admission interview. This is an essential process which will continue throughout the individual's hospital stay and during outpatient follow-up treatment as well. Initially, people entering the hospital often have goals which are vague (e.g., "I want to be normal like everyone else"), unhealthy (e.g., a person already underweight may want to "lose ten more pounds of fat"), or unrealistic (e.g., to be "cured" in six weeks). In our program we continually challenge people to set healthy goals that are "S.M.A.R.T." (i.e., Specific, Measurable, Attainable, Realistic, and Trackable). Initially, many patients have great difficulty doing this. They may resist setting S.M.A.R.T. goals as a way of holding onto their illness and avoiding the discomfort that inevitably accompanies change; or they may have little experience with the process of setting and achieving goals. Goal-setting is also made difficult by the eating-disordered person's lack of trust in the process of cooperative problem-solving and by their sense of personal inadequacy and shame which we discussed earlier in chapter 3. We will have more to say about goal-setting later in this chapter when we discuss therapeutic contracting. The important point here is that we see S.M.A.R.T. goal-setting as essential to successful treatment, and we therefore encourage and teach the establishment of healthy goals from the outset.

Finally, the initial evaluation includes an assessment of the patient's family of origin and current social support system. This process also begins with the pre-admission interview, during which basic information is obtained both from the perspective patient and from the family members who accompany her. After meeting together in a group, family members are sometimes interviewed separately by the social worker to facilitate the information-gathering process. From the beginning, we stress the importance of family involvement, begin to educate family members concerning eating disorders, assess the family's role in the patient's illness, and assess the capacity of family members to support the patient's recovery.

In summary, the initial evaluation encompasses the physical, psychological, behavioral, and social aspects of the patient's life. It begins with the pre-admission interview and is the primary objective during the patient's first two weeks in the hospital. The evaluation provides the information essential for planning the therapy that will follow.

### The Treatment Team

As we have mentioned previously, the eating-disorders treatment team consists of a psychiatrist (Dr. Swift), a social worker, a program coordinator (K. Zraly), the art and dance therapists, and designated members of the hospital's nursing staff. Although our roles overlap considerably, each of us has distinct functions and responsibilities.

In our program the psychiatrist sees patients for an initial psychiatric evaluation and meets frequently with each patient throughout their treatment to assess their progress. Decisions regarding medications are made by the psychiatrist. The psychiatrist also sees patients for individual psychotherapy sessions and co-leads, with the program coordinator, a twice-weekly therapeutic contracting group.

The social worker sees each patient during the initial evaluation period for the purpose of obtaining a detailed psychosocial history. This is an account of the patient's life which focuses largely on the quality of her interpersonal relationships and her feelings about herself and others. The social worker also meets with family members to gather information about the patient, and to get a better understanding of the patient's past and current social environment. When indicated, the social worker sees the patient and family members together for family therapy. Finally, the social worker sees all patients in the program twice weekly for group therapy sessions which focus primarily on family issues and the patient's relationships with parents, spouse, children, siblings, etc.

The program coordinator is the person responsible for maintaining good communication between treatment team members and for transmitting information back and forth between patients and the team. Treatment team decisions regarding privileges, passes, and schedule changes, etc., are communicated to the patient by the program coordinator. Similarly, patients' requests, complaints, etc., are brought to the treatment team by the program coordinator. In short, the program coordinator ensures that nothing "falls between the cracks," and that treatment staff are kept up-to-date and are coordinated in their approach to each patient. In addition, the program coordinator is the primary person who deals with the patient's issues regarding food and weight. Meal-planning and nutrition education are the responsibility of the program coordinator, with assistance from the hospital dietician. The program coordinator weighs each patient weekly and sees patients individually to explore issues regarding their bodies, their eating behaviors, the significance of their eating-disorder symptoms, and ways of giving up their symptoms in favor of more functional behavior. When indicated, the program coordinator negotiates behavioral contracts with individual patients regarding weight and relevant eating behaviors.

The program coordinator also takes patients off grounds for a weekly food-shopping trip and subsequently supervises "food lab," during which the patients prepare a meal for themselves. She co-leads with the psychiatrist a twice-weekly therapeutic contracting group. Finally, she participates in team meetings, keeps statistical data, orders books and other supplies used in the program, and arranges transportation for patients attending off-grounds group meetings such as Al-Anon, ACoA, or O.A.

In many ways the nursing staff are the most important part of the treatment team. Nurses have more contact with patients than other members of the team, and therefore more opportunity to have constructive therapeutic impact. In our program, nurses are expected to be co-therapists, not merely people who carry out orders and make observations of patient behaviors. Through their participation in weekly treatment team meetings, and both formal and informal in-service training, interested nurses are taught and encouraged to take an active role in the treatment process. It is a nurse who is most likely to be present when a patient's symptoms are most obvious. Bingeing, purging, refusing to eat, inappropriate social behavior, displays of strong emotion, self-injurious behavior, withdrawal, and self-isolation are usually first observed by nursing personnel. Effective intervention by nursing staff when these behaviors first occur can be of more value to the patient than discussing the behavior with a therapist hours or days later. In our program nurses have wide latitude to meet with patients individually or in groups on a scheduled or impromptu basis to deal with any problem they feel comfortable addressing.

The hospital dietician acts as an advisor to both patients and staff regarding dietary matters. Patients requiring special diets for weight reduction or the management of medical problems meet with the dietician for meal-planning. In concert with the program coordinator, the dietician provides patients with information about healthy meal-planning.

The art therapist meets twice weekly with patients in our program. Through a variety of structured and unstructured activities, the patients are given opportunities to experience and express feelings through drawing, painting, collage, and other media. The dance therapist also meets twice a week with our patients, utilizing mime, charades, dance, and other non-verbal techniques which encourage patients to become more aware of their bodies, their feelings, and their capacity to communicate through body movement.

## Schedule of Activities

As rapidly as possible, patients in our program are phased into a full schedule of activities which provide them with a diversified range of therapeutic activities. The complete eating-disorder program schedule is given in Appendix D. Much of the schedule is self-explanatory, but a few activities deserve further explanation.

*Therapeutic Contracting.* The therapeutic contracting group, which meets on Tuesday and Friday afternoons, is co-led by the psychiatrist and program coordinator. In this group patients discuss long-term and short-term goals and define specific goals for the coming week. Each patient's goals are examined by the entire group to ensure that they are S.M.A.R.T. (specific, measurable, attainable, relevant, trackable). During subsequent contracting sessions each patient's progress toward achieving her goals is assessed. If a patient has suceeded in achieving goals from the previous week, new goals are set. If she was unable to achieve her goals, the obstacles are identified and new goals are set which address those obstacles. For example, a patient dealing with long-repressed feelings about childhood events decided that she would share her feelings with her mother during her mother's next visit. When her mother came to visit, however, the patient found herself paralyzed by fear and was unable to carry out her plan. During the following contracting session, she revised her contract and agreed to write a letter to her mother instead. Although writing the letter also evoked considerable fear, she was able to do it with support from the group. Her letter broke the ice and later she was able to share more of her feelings during conversations with her mother.

We have found that having patients set S.M.A.R.T. goals on a weekly basis greatly speeds the recovery process. As is true of most of us, eating-disordered people find it easier to talk about their problems than to do something about them. Talking, after all, is a low-risk activity. Doing is much more risky, and many people, especially people who feel inadequate or ashamed, find it very difficult to carry out even relatively simple goals like "reading ten pages in my workbook," or "going to morning exercise every day next week." Effective therapeutic contracting rapidly brings patients face-to-face with the internal obstacles (feelings and beliefs) they must deal with in order for recovery to proceed.

*Shopping and Food Lab.* Grocery stores and kitchens are difficult places for most eating-disordered people. Typically, being in such places triggers eating-disordered behavior. The ambivalence discussed in chapter 4 is often evoked by entering areas where food is present. Patients often experience intense anxiety, impulses to binge, or impulses to run away. The weekly shopping trip and food lab give patients an opportunity to face these feelings in a context which offers protection and support. The program coordinator takes the patients food-shopping and then supervises the subsequent preparation of a meal. The dietician often assists, especially if the group is large. This activity thus provides for practical experience in meal-planning and nutrition education, desensitization to stores and kitchens, and a wealth of subjective experience which can be explored in both group and individual therapy sessions.

*Playing with Food.* Occasionally we vary the weekly shopping and food lab in the following way. The patients are taken to the grocery store as usual, but upon arriving at the store, they are told to disregard their shopping list and instead are each given ten dollars and told to spend it all on their favorite foods. A multitude of emotional responses often result from this unexpected change of plan, and brief "crisis counseling" on the part of accompanying staff is sometimes required. After making their purchases, the patients return to the hospital and are taken to a room which has been largely cleared of furniture except for a plastic sheet which covers the floor. They are then told that for the next hour they and members of the eating-disorders team will play with the food. Again, a wide range of responses is usually elicited. Most patients experience initial anxiety and resist the idea of using food as a medium for play. One of our patients became extremely anxious and retreated to a corner where she sat sobbing in a fetal position. With support from team members and co-patients, these initial impulses to run are overcome. In fact, we have never had a patient fail to join in eventually. Sleeves are rolled up, aprons are donned by some, and soon staff and patients alike are actively involved in creating a giant finger painting of food. Castles, rivers, mountains, and valleys are sculpted. M & Ms become the eyes and noses of cupcake people. Playful food fights occur. Balls are formed from the mishmash of dozens of different foods and used as bombs or for playing catch with other group members. Foods ranging from chocolate syrup and ice cream to pretzels and hard candy become an amorphous mass on the floor. Playful, hostile, cooperative, and competitive impulses are expressed. Everyone has fun and some get pretty messy. The scene is similar to a group building and destroying sand castles at the beach. Eventually everyone towels off and the entire mess, plastic sheet, food, and towels, are ceremoniously disposed of in a dumpster by the entire group.

This event can have powerful and useful effects. From this activity patients can begin to experience their power over food.

The idea that food can be fun and can enhance inter-personal relationships is novel to many eating-disordered patients. The feelings and thoughts triggered by this experience are often a useful source of insight and self-awareness. We have found that this activity is useful in that it helps us to better understand our patients, and that it helps patients to better understand themselves, too.

### Family Therapy

Family therapy is an integral piece of the recovery process. During hospitalization we engage the family (when feasible) from the outset. The family meets with the social worker, preferably on a weekly basis, to begin to process out how the eating-disordered person and her behavior have affected the family system. It's important to remember that each family member is entitled to express his or her thoughts and feelings. Very often, families experience a sense of needing to hold these feelings in, fearing that if they were to express them, the eating-disordered person might get upset. But whether they are a parent, sibling or spouse, each family member will inevitably have feelings toward the patient and toward other family members. Family therapy encourages the open sharing of such feelings.

Throughout family therapy there is an identification of the roles that each member has taken on. A primary goal of family therapy is the identification of these roles, and how they either hinder or enhance family relationships. Like the eating-disordered person who has spent most of her life fantasizing about a "Brady Bunch type of family," initially the family see themselves in the same way. A common comment we hear is, "Doesn't every family have problems?" We respond with "more than likely." What needs to be understood is that the eating-disordered person comes from a dysfunctional family. Most often the family members exhibit some of the same issues we've presented throughout the book—issues dealing with difficulty expressing feelings and issues with control. These all need to be addressed with the family.

Family therapy seems to go in two directions: either the family is resistant to looking at the fact that there is a problem, or the family feels that they need to "fix" the eating-disordered person.

Another issue which most always surfaces is "What do we do with the eating part of the disorder?" Our suggestion is to stay out of the food issues. Sometimes this presents a seemingly impossible task. It is difficult when, in the case of the anorexic, meal-time becomes like a battle zone. It's hard to watch a family member refuse to eat without getting into power struggles and trying to force them to eat. Getting the anorexic to willingly engage herself in therapy can be like moving a mountain. Everyone around her must try not to give her any choices. Obviously, she is going through a difficult, painful time but it also becomes evident that her ability to make healthy choices is seriously impaired. With the bulimic and compulsive overeater, it may be equally as frustrating. It is frustrating to have gone grocery shopping for an entire week's worth of food only to find that most of it has been consumed within twenty-four hours. This needs to be confronted, and boundaries need to be established. Unfortunately, the eating-disordered person will most often deny that she has eaten any of the missing food. It's very easy to fall into power struggles with eating-disorderd people.

We feel it is important to confront these issues in a direct but supportive way: "I love you very much, but I'm angry that all the food is missing. What are we going to do about this?"

Family work is essential. For whatever reason, the family

constellation has provided a nesting ground for some unhealthy thoughts, feelings, and behaviors. Remember, the feelings of family members are fully as important as the feelings of the eating-disordered person.

*Off-Grounds Activities.* Many of our patients participate in therapeutic activities outside of the hospital. This depends upon the need and interest of each individual. Patients struggling with alcohol and/or drug abuse problems are generally scheduled to attend evening or weekend A.A. or N.A. meetings when their condition has stabilized sufficiently. Some of these meetings take place at the hospital, but many are held off-grounds. Patients from alcoholic families frequently attend Al-Anon or ACoA groups. Others, especially people with overweight bulimia or compulsive overeating, find O.A. a useful resource. Although our eating-disorders program is not a Twelve Step program, we borrow liberally from the Twelve Step model and encourage many of our patients to become actively involved in such programs.

### Progressing Through the Program

Patients begin their inpatient treatment by being admitted to the locked unit. Initially they have little freedom of movement and few privileges. Meals are prescribed, access to food is strictly controlled, and bathrooms are locked for two hours following meals. By the time they are ready for discharge they are living on the hospital's open unit, have free access to food and bathrooms, can come and go around the hospital without supervivson, are participating in off-grounds activities, and have had several passes at home. The rate at which an individual progresses through the program is determined by how well she handles each new responsibility.

For most patients, eating in the central patient dining room is a major challenge. There, access to food is relatively unrestricted. Patients often experience strong impulses to binge and considerable anxiety, even though they begin by eating only one meal per day (usually breakfast) off the unit. Another frequent crisis point is when a patient begins going out of the hospital for day passes with friends or family. Often old conflicts are revived and maladaptive behaviors are triggered by returning home and spending unstructured time with other people outside the protective environment of the hospital. Relapses are fairly common at both of these junctures. Understanding and overcoming the causes of such relapses then becomes a major focus of both individual and family therapy. Whenever possible we help our patients to deal with their anxieties and relapses without taking away hard-won privileges, but at times this is not possible or safe. Generally patients tell us when they need more protection, and only infrequently have we had to suspend privileges over the objections of a patient.

### Discharge Planning

Arranging for continued outpatient treatment and other support necessary to continue the recovery process is a required part of every patient's therapeutic contract. As recovery progresses and discharge approaches, this becomes increasingly important. Inpatient treatment provides the foundation for eventual recovery, but unless the individual continues in treatment after leaving the hospital, relapse is a virtual certainty. Even with intense outpatient follow-up, relapses may occur. Therefore, we begin to explore outpatient resources soon after admission and engage patients and family in discharge planning well in advance of the patient's actual discharge date.

Since many eating-disordered people have become relatively isolated and disconnected from healthy sources of social and emotional support, discharge planning is a major task for some patients. As is true for alcoholics and drug-addicted people, changes in social activities, friend-ships, and living arrangements may be called for. The people, places, and things that trigger symptomatic be-havior should be modified as much as possible. Depending upon individual needs, patients may decide to join new social or recreational groups, change jobs (restaurant work is definitely contraindicated!), change living arrange-ments, or end unhealthy relationships. Adequate outpa-tient therapy may include individual and/or group psychotherapy, O.A., ACoA or other Twelve Step pro-grams, continuation of medication, or referral to a support group for people with eating disorders. When patients come to us on referral from outside therapists, part of their discharge plan will ordinarily be to resume treatment with that therapist. When they have no outside therapist we continue to work with them as outpatients when pos-sible, or assist them in locating suitable resources near their home. Often patients are given passes so they can meet with a new therapist or attend a group meeting once or twice prior to discharge, in order to smooth the transi-tion from hospital to home. When the patient is returning to a previous therapist or being referred to a new one, that therapist is encouraged to meet with the patient and treat-ment team prior to discharge to discuss the patient's needs and ensure continuity of treatment.

### Treatment Philosophy

In all our interactions with eating-disordered patients, we strive to address the core issues which underlie their symptoms. Symptoms are by no means discounted or ig-nored, but any confrontation of symptoms or restriction of activity is done out of concern for the well-being of the patient, rather than because the symptoms themselves are "bad" or "not allowed." If a patient is known to have binged or purged or hidden food, an attempt is made to help her to identify three things: First, the basic impulse underlying the behavior; second, the maladaptive beliefs that blocked healthy expression of the impulse; third, constructive, healthy options for expressing the impulse. For example, an anorexic patient began skipping meals after a home visit with her family. If this behavior were to persist or endanger the patient's health we might respond by suspending home visits and having the patient eat her meals on the unit under close supervision. However, our ultimate objective was to understand what had happened. In this instance, the patient was able to recognize that she had felt hurt and angry when her family failed to give her the attention she wanted. She was afraid to ask for attention for fear of angering them and driving them further away. She dealt with the conflict by fasting. Several dysfunctional beliefs were identified. These included: (1) "If I express my needs people will leave me," (2) "I can't make it if my family leaves me," (3) "I shouldn't get angry," and finally (4) "This whole mess is all my fault." After unraveling this chain of events her eating improved, and in this instance, no restricton of privileges was necessary.

In our dealings with patients we attempt to model a cooperative problem-solving approach. Surface behaviors and symptoms are confronted only when they can be identified as self-defeating to the patient and/or contrary to the welfare of others. In fact, it can usually be demonstrated that behavior contrary to the welfare of others *is self-defeating* as well, so almost all confrontation can be made from a position of caring about the best interests of the patient.

Through our emphasis on group therapy and group activities we build a mini-community within the hospital, which encourages mutual support and cooperation between patients and discourages competitive interactions. Underlying everything else, we believe that people have an innate biological drive to grow and to develop more and better ways of coping with the vicissitudes of life. Our experience has been that given an environment which is supportive of non-judgmental self-awareness, assertive expression of thoughts and feelings, and cooperative problem-solving, people will make significant progress along the road to recovery.

# 6

## Drowning In A Sea Of Fear

"**S**ometimes I feel like I'm drowning," a patient once told me. "It feels as though I finally managed to get my head above all this stuff long enough to catch my breath and before I know it, I feel like someone or something has come along and dunked me—far enough down that it seems like forever until I get the next breath." "Drowning in what?" I asked. She responded with the ever-familiar "I don't know." "Fear," I suggested. After a moment, she began to cry. "Yeah," she said, "That's exactly what it feels like—like I'm drowning in a sea of fear."

In the first few chapter we have explored the personality characteristics and core issues of the eating-disordered person. Now we would like to examine the difficult areas and issues the person is faced with throughout the course of recovery.

Most eating-disordered people enter therapy with a strong sense of ambivalence. For most, problems with eating have been long-term, and the thought of living life without an eating disorder becomes not only a frightening thought, but also a seemingly unreal one. Giving up their eating disorder becomes the same as giving up their identity.

To date, we have not had an anorexic walk into our office and say, "I can't stand this any more, I need help." Most often they are accompanied by a family member or friend who is at their wits' end as to how to help this person. As was mentioned in the introduction, the typical response is "Why is everyone so up in arms? I just lost a few pounds." The anorexic has found an identity within the eating disorder. The fear involved with acknowledging that a problem exists far outweighs the reality. (In speaking with the eating-disordered person who is well into the recovery process it becomes more clear that an awareness of the unhealthy position they were in existed all along). Denial becomes the single most difficult issue with the anorexic. Denial, for all intents and purposes, is the defense mechanism which enables the patient to avoid dealing with the fear involved in looking at herself from the inside out. The fear that they will not be accepted, approved of, or loved unless they are thin is paralyzing.

Bulimics most often seek treatment on their own. As they sit in the office recounting the years of bingeing and purging, there is a strong sense of guilt and remorse. Most bulimics have been able to carry on a seemingly "normal" life with little hint that something is wrong. By the time a bulimic seeks out treatment she has had just about all she can take with this eating disorder.

Most bulimics will state that they are unclear as to whether they want to give up this disorder, but are clear in stating that they are mentally and physically exhausted from it. Like the anorexic, the bulimic has made this her identity. She finds it difficult to imagine life without it. Bulimia out of the three disorders is probably the most difficult to own for two reasons. One, the bulimic's weight does not signify that there is any difficulty inside or out, whereas the anorexic has a thin or emaciated body and the compulsive overeater has the heavier or obese body. Two, although starving or overeating are not condoned both seem to be viewed in a more understanding manner than eating and throwing up.

Compulsive overeaters most often get caught in a whirl-wind of "diets" and "miracle cures" to target their behavior of eating. They recognize they are overeating and often will only allow themselves to concentrate on getting their eating straightened out. This is not to say that the compulsive overeater does not seek treatment; but usually there is an underlying panic to "fix" the eating first. It is not unusual that as compulsive overeaters skip from diet to diet they also skip from therapist to therapist. Once they realize the therapist cannot fix them, and may ask them to look at underlying reasons for the overeating, compulsive overeaters seek out another way to lose weight.

Eating disorders work for the patient. It is the fear of giving up something that works, that keeps the eating disorder going. How do they work? With all three of the above-mentioned disorders the common thread—whether the person is obsessing about how to get out of eating for the day, or about how to get rid of the food they just binged on, or about how and what kinds of food are available to eat throughout the day—is that the focus on food, weight, and meals is so consuming that it distracts and de-focuses from other thoughts and feelings that may be causing pain, discomfort, or confusion. Think of eating disorders as a circle. At the top of the circle is worrying—a trait that the eating-disordered person has excelled at throughout her existence. This constant worrying produces anxiety. (Allow yourself to remember the last time you became anxious about something. You may have gotten a headache, your muscles may have ached, or you may have experienced an overall sense of physical tension that made you feel as if you needed to go out running or scribble all over a piece of paper. Regardless, you recognized you needed to alleviate the tension.) It is at this point of relieving the physical tension created by anxiety that the eating disorder is called upon.

For the anorexic it is not the actual food that appears to relieve the tension, but the obsessive consuming thoughts about how to lose another pound, or the intense desire to compulsively exercise. For most humans, exercise can and does alleviate tension. They exercise until they feel some-what more relaxed and in control, and can then look at whatever was creating the anxiety. It is important to point out that exercise, for the anorexic, serves as a way to de-focus and distract herself from dealing with whatever is causing her this anxiety.

When the bulimic becomes anxious, the thoughts of bingeing usually increase quickly. When feelings start to surface, the bulimic becomes uncomfortable and fright-ened by those feelings. (In chapter 3, we discussed the difficult nature of allowing themselves to experience feel-ings—"It's not-OK to feel.") The feelings are experienced as being pushed up from inside and threatening to spill out. Before the expression of these feelings actually comes out, she has begun a binge. As the food goes in, it pushes the feelings back down and out of the way. As the binge continues, the person's focus has now shifted from uncom-fortable feelings to physical discomfort from the ingesting of a large quantity of food. Now, the only issues the person allows herself to experience is the guilt from eating all the food, and the overpowering need to get rid of the food through purging. Once the purge is completed the person returns to worrying, which will eventually lead her to become anxious once again. As with the anorexic, the process serves as a way to distract and de-focus from dealing with feelings.

Compulsive overeaters are similar to the bulimic, except they do not purge. The use of food as emotional comfort appears to stem from early life. If they weren't feeling well, the message became, "Have something to eat, you'll feel better." If they were sad the message was, "Don't be sad, go fix yourself something to eat." The compulsive overeater learned early on that no matter what uncomfort-able feeling they were experiencing, food would fix it. Again, as with the anorexic and bulimic it became a way to distract and de-focus from whatever was causing them this discomfort. Remember earlier in the chapter, it was discussed that most humans recognize the need to alleviate the tension first; then they feel more relaxed to problem-solve. Unfortunately, because the eating disorder is so consuming they never allow themselves to return to whatever was creating the anxiety and effectively problem-solve.

Short-term, the eating disorder works for the patient. The bingeing or starving temporarily makes the person feel better. The food or power she feels over it becomes her best friend—she can call on it any time. It doesn't argue or talk back and it's very reliable. Long-term, it is debilitating. Eating disorders are one of the most complex disorders to wrk with. Most patients are looking for a guarantee: "If I give this up you have to *promise* me everything will be OK and will work out." To date, we know of no guarantees.

If we take a look back on the outside-in theory, it becomes clear that eating-disorder persons are "re-acters," rather than "pro-acters." They will revolve their lives around others even if it means compromising their own belief system. They are people who fear their own feelings. Very often we encounter people in therapy who can express very clearly how they feel about an incident that may have created discomfort for them. When asked if they shared how they felt with the other person involved they said, "Oh no, I could never let that person know how I feel, they might get mad." It becomes quickly evident, then, that what is being said to that other person most often does not match the patient's true feelings. Revealing their feelings is their primary fear, and seems to occur most often in intimate relationships.

When most eating-disordered people enter therapy, a prominent fear is that we will take the eating disorder from them. One of the first and clearest messages we give them is that we do not want to take their eating disorder away, but we would like to help them address their fears and develop healthy coping mechanisms. We also let them know that if they cannot, throughout the course of therapy, establish other ways of dealing with their fears they can keep the eating disorder.

The reality is that no one can take away their eating disorder because they possess it, they control it. What they choose not to look at is that by seeking treatment, they have taken the first step in the process of letting go, not only of their eating disorders, but also of their fears.

The eating disorder serves as a cover-up. In most circumstances the patients we see come from a dysfunctional family system. Most often, as parents were fighting or discussions were being held, the message was "everything is OK, go back to your room," or "everything is not-OK; maybe when you're older we'll tell you more about it." Our experience has been that this is when fear becomes incorporated into the child's thinking process. In the first message, the child sees that there is something wrong, yet is being told that everything is OK. In the second message, the child learns something *is* wrong but that she is too young to understand. Both messages leave the child with feelings of not being able to handle issues. In turn, the child begins to question whether something is wrong with her—that she cannot handle a difficult situation. She grows up with the fear that something bad is going to happen, the fear that she's not-OK, and the fear that she may be abandoned if something is wrong.

On the opposite end of the spectrum is the message of, "You can handle everything and anything." We have found that many of our patients have learned to listen to one or the other parent's problems at an early age. The child becomes the therapist, the emotional support system. Here is where she learns to become the caretaker and protector.

Take, for example, the case of Sally, mentioned in chapter 3. Sally often found herself intervening between her mom and dad when her dad would drink. She feared for her mother's safety (protector), as well as becoming her emotional support system (caretaker). Sally perceived and quite honestly believed that during these times her mother was unable to handle the situation, so she would step in and take care of it. After a while, Sally was unable to distinguish when and where her mother could handle a crisis, so Sally learned to handle all of them all of the time. The more anger Sally felt toward her father, the more protective she became of her mother.

Sally learned that she needed to become everything that her father was supposed to be as a husband, short of being her mother's lover. This is not to blame her mother, but to understand more clearly how the eating-disordered person develops patterns of thinking. So Sally continued doing her "job" taking care of people, and eventually found herself doing nothing but that. What makes this a difficult issue is that the eating-disordered person never allows a sense of self to fully develop. She begins to miss out on after-school activities, hurrying home to make sure everything is OK. She wants to include her mother in all her social engagements, feeling sorry that her mother's own have fallen apart. She becomes a mature, responsible adult—on the outside. Inside, she is a mess. She constantly worries and is unable to really enjoy things, fearing she may be needed at home at any minute. One of the messages, discussed earlier, is that it is not-OK to have her own needs and feelings. As the child is experiencing feelings regarding the home situation, most often she finds it difficult, if not impossible, to let anyone know what's going on inside her.

In an alcoholic or dysfunctional family, the child is told, "Whatever goes on in this house stays within these four walls." The message again states, "Everything is really not-OK, but you're not allowed to share the feelings you may be experiencing with anyone else." This in turn sets up a demand upon the child to present the "outside" (family life) as fine.

The child who learns to swallow her feelings brings this trait into adolescence, when feelings become more confusing and difficult. She begins to experience anger and a sense of emptiness. Both feelings generate from her own needs not being met. She may feel unsupported by other siblings or family members in her quest to make everything OK. What begins to occur is that the feelings are turned inward, toward the self. "Maybe I can't handle it, maybe I am worthless, why would anyone like me, and if they did like me they wouldn't after they found out what I'm really like inside." All of the messages she perceived as a child are now being validated and reinforced. What makes it more difficult is that most people view her as "happy, peppy, and bursting with love." So she begins to live in her own world, tormented by this voice which is always doubting and questioning her worth as a person. Eventually, the tension created by the two worlds snaps. It is at this point that the eating disorder gets started. For most, it is not a conscious decision to abuse food, but one that takes on value gradually, like the alcoholic who starts out with one social drink and ends up drinking continuously.

Fear becomes her number one enemy. Since the message she has come to believe is that she is incapable of handling issues, she lives in fear of everything. Our experiences has been that most eating-disordered people don't learn anything new about themselves throughout the course of therapy. What they do begin to realize is that fourteen tons of brick, each brick representing some kind of fear, is weighing them down. Their instinct (gut level) tells them to confront, to be honest, to trust, but the fear of rejection, conflict, and abandonment keeps them feeling trapped and helpless. We have had many patients say, "I know what I need to do, I just can't get myself to do it." Facing and dealing with their fears takes time, patience and understanding on the part of therapists and patients alike. We can't help but mention that this is one of the most frustrating components in therapy. The therapist knows the patient will be OK, feel better, and maybe even believe in herself a little more but she needs to experience it in her own space and time. When she begins to let go of her fears she also begins to let go of her eating disorder. Once she confronts her fears, the purpose served by the eating disorder loses its value. When a patient relapses and begins to hide behind the eating disorder once again, one of the first questions we address is "What are you afraid of?" When she owns that fear, the recovery process continues.

When the fear becomes too intense, the eating-disordered person begins to create a world of fantasy. This world cannot hurt her. It allows the eating-disordered person to create a warm, secure, fear-free environment. Unfortunately, she begins to believe it is reality. In the next chapter we will explore the fork in the road; that point at which the eating-disordered person must choose her life in the fantasy or her life in the reality.

# 7

## The Fork In the Road

A famous singer back in the 1970s wrote a song about coming to a fork in the road. He sang about knowing his choices were clear, but the fear of not knowing which way to go was stifling. He saw one road as simpler—an acceptance of life; the other road offered final peace. When he chose the road of acceptance of life his vision became his relief.

Throughout life we are all faced with different forks in the road. As children, we encounter the different stages of development. It is at these stages, or forks, that we begin to formulate who we are. An infant must learn to trust her mother for feeding, changing, and nurturing. If this does not develop, the infant withdraws into a depressive state. She learns to mistrust that her needs will be met on demand. As a toddler, she begins to experiment with her autonomy, learning self-control without the loss of self-esteem and rightful dignity. If she fears this autonomy, she will develop feelings of shame and doubt. She will suffer from a low self-esteem, a sense of secretiveness, and feelings of persecution. The preschooler learns to take initiative over her life. She learns to be loving, relaxed, energetic, and task-oriented. If she becomes uncomfortable with these issues, a sense of guilt overtakes her. She develops the ability to deny, and feels paralyzed and inhibited and begins to overcompensate for these feelings by showing off. This is when the child also complains of feeling sick all the time or injures herself quite often.

As the child becomes school-aged she experiences the need to be productive. She develops a good attention span, sticks with tasks, and becomes more comfortable working with different instruments. If these feelings become inhibited, the child begins to sense feelings of being inferior. She feels inadequate, and from this inadequacy she learns to conform to what others are doing and her sense of self begins to break down. During her adolescent years she begins to establish an identity and a level of confidence. If the other stages continue to be unhealthy she experiences confusion in who she is. She begins to act-out and over-identify with heroes, cliques, and crowds. She has given up her sense of self, feeling that others are much better.

In the young adult the most common issue becomes intimacy. It is at this time that the healthy individual who has established a sense of self begins to learn how to make a commitment, to sacrifice and compromise, and to feel more comfortable in sexual relations. For those whose pattern has been compounded by unhealthy development, there is a sense of isolation. They become distant and self-absorbed and they begin to exhibit character problems.

If the child experiences failure in any of these stages, she is likely to have greater difficulty achieving success in future stages of development. If we review what has been written so far, it becomes increasingly clear that the eating-disorder person exhibits most, if not all, of the unhealthy developmental characteristics.

Many people have asked, "Why does an eating disorder start most often in adolescence? Consider the maladaptive level of functioning across all the stages. By the time the child has reached adolescence, the combination and over-lapping of these stages has created a weakened, insecure, frightened person. Why food for some people, alcohol and drugs for others, we're not sure. The end result is that food serves to distract and to de-focus from other painful areas.

Entering therapy becomes one of the most difficult tasks the person with an eating disorder will face. We have explored the fear attached to this endeavor, but the real resistance maintains itself in the face of actually acknowledging that a problem severe enough to warrant therapy exists.

Most often, therapy is initiated by a major crisis in a person's life, be it the breakup of a meaningful relationship, or the threat of losing a job; with any crisis, the eating disorder almost always plays a significant role.

So yet another fork: whether to seek treatment or not. Our experience has been that this fork may be encountered more than once or twice. She may initiate therapy but become too frightened to continue once issues outside of the major crisis are addressed. It is not unusual, albeit frustrating, for the individual to hop from therapist to therapist, just as she did from diet to diet. Some have gotten so out of control with their feelings and behaviors that they welcome therapy and commit to it; others need more time to flounder about looking for the "miracle cure." Regardless, when an individual commits herself to therapy she has taken the first, and sometimes most difficult, step toward recovery.

Most of us are faced with different forks almost every day. Hopefully, we weigh out the pros and cons and make the best, healthiest decision we can. Decision. That becomes the key factor in moving ahead. Since the eating-disordered person has acquired most of her validation from the outside-in, it becomes overwhelming when she is faced with a decision—especially if it involves another person. Most people with eating disorders allow others to set the pace.

It has been our experience that when an eating-disordered person initially enters therapy, it is important to focus in on whatever immediate crisis is going on in her life. She will resist going back into her younger years searching for the reason(s) she has an eating disorder. Anyone who has ever worked with or been around a person with an eating disorder quickly acquires an understanding of the words "instantaneous gratification"—they want it fixed, over and done with yesterday. One of the questions asked with quickness and intensity is, "How long am I going to have to be in therapy?" When we respond with, "It's hard to say—we feel anything less than six months to a year would be selling yourself short," there is a look of "You mean you can't fix this by next week?" Many, understandably, are so caught up in the moment that they fail to recognize the eating disorder as only a symptom of many issues accumulated throughout the years.

Although we explored the different stages of development, it is important to remember that you need to work backward with a person with an eating disorder. It is important that they begin working on whatever fork they feel they are facing now. Most, if not all, have high standards and set unattainable goals at the beginning. It is here they need to feel, see, and experience any progress possible.

We have seen how people with eating disorders have difficulty with issues such as low self-esteem, assertiveness, and levels of confidence. It becomes apparent throughout treatment that when the person is faced with becoming more assertive or increasing her level of self-confidence, she has reached a fork in the road. The eating-disordered person may struggle for weeks or months, playing out every possible scenario before deciding which road to choose. Very often she would like the therapist to make the decision for her. This can be a frustraing crossroad for the therapist, since certainly the therapist knows that the healthier choice will allow the person to be one step closer to recovery. The forks encountered can range from emotionally intense (letting go of a relationship) to minimal thought ("should I allow myself to have an extra spoonful of something"). Regardless of the intensity, the forks are very real and painful for the eating-disordered person.

Recently we had a session with one of our patients (Kaylee) whom we sometimes see together. She became tearful during the session, and when asked what was behind the tears she replied, "Anger." She stated she was angry with both of us for not acknowledging the intense emotional pain she had been experiencing for the last six months. She stated she was even more angry that we had not been able to "fix" this pain. We both glanced at each other, mentally searching through the issues addressed within the last six months. Finally, one of us spoke up admitting the difficulty in pinpointing where this intense pain was coming from. Having worked with her for over two years, we were both experiencing feelings of discomfort for missing something so important. She went on to explain that within the last few months she had been experiencing tremendous turmoil. She described herself sitting at a fork in the road. One road she had spent most—if not all—of her life traveling. This was the road of dreams. Dreams of how her life *could* be different; *wishing* for happiness and inner peace. This road allowed her to fantasize about "a Brady Bunch" type of lifestyle, where family members communicated and worked through difficult times, where people were respectful of one another and where people showed signs of love and affection.

Then there was the other road. The one that represented reality. "This is the road," she said, "where no matter how much I allow myself to fantasize, my mind always brings me back to the way my life really is." She perceived her life as a continuous crisis and felt that even when she allowed herself to deal with the turmoil, something else was always waiting in the wings. As painful as she experienced the realities to be, she was also clear in describing what they were. She felt as though she had to be the responsible child.

Kaylee was the oldest of four children. Her father was an alcoholic who went on week-long binges, something resulting in both verbal and physical abuse. Her mother vacillated between being emotionally needy and being overcontrolling. She often found herself as a small child physically intervening between her mother and father as they were fighting. She discovered that if she was able to make as much noise as she could, or create as much commotion as she could, her parents would eventually focus in on her and stop fighting. Unfortunately, her plan of attack worked. So she became the identified deterrent. On the other hand, she also experienced feelings of needing to protect her younger brothers and sister. Once her parents stopped fighting she would go in to calm her siblings down, making up all kinds of excuses as to why mom and dad fought a lot.

She began to experience intense confusion. As mom would get her ready for school she would say, "Now, what went on last night between your father and me is not to be talked about with anybody once you walk out the front door." Kaylee began to feel a sense of shame and embarrassment that her parents would argue so much, while at the same time she felt a strong sense of loyalty, and responsibility for keeping family secrets. So the internal conflict begins.

As an adult, she mastered the art of hiding her feelings. Her parents promoted the message "Go out and pretend that this family is fine," and she modeled the same. On the outside she presented the nice, caring, sensitive person— on the inside she was in constant pain, carrying with her the message learned long ago, "It's not-OK to feel."

It's important to understand that Kaylee began to minimize the significance of her own feelings. It was more important to make sure everyone else was OK. She also experienced the reality of how much time she felt had been wasted because of the role she played in the family. She recognized the constant anxiety and the fact that this anxiety took away from her focusing on herself and her own needs. Another reality was owning the fact that she needed to break the bond of taking care of her mother, or dealing with her father's behaviors. The difficulty wasn't so much the realization of these issues, but the continuous struggle toward not feeling as though she was abandoning them, or letting go of keeping everything in check. The realization that she was now in a recovery process was one of the most difficult. She experienced this as a sense of failure: "I did all this work, I kept everything going, and now I'm the one who has to surrender by going to therapy."

Although these feelings of realizations were difficult, she also stated she experienced a sense of acceptance and ownership. She needed to accept that her schooling was put off because she couldn't concentrate on school, and that her role was not to get ahead in her own life, but to always take care of the family. She needed to accept that the family was not the "Brady Bunch"; that the reality was that she was the product of a severely dysfunctional family.

Once the realities were identified, she was left with many uncomfortable feelings. She experienced a tremendous sense of sadness that the family life had lost its worth. The most prevalent feeling is that of anger toward her parents. She felt a though they should have been there to guide her through healthy development. The reality was that they were not.

When Kaylee finished relaying to us what it was that she had been experiencing, the three of us began to take a look at the positive steps she had taken by sharing her feelings. First, because she had learned it's not-OK to feel, she was credited with the ability to share these feelings with us. We pointed out that in order for her to get angry with us she had to have established a significant bond of trust. One of her biggest fears, learned early on, was, "I can't let you know I'm angry with you because you may get mad and abandon me." She needed to know that we were not going to leave. She also expressed anger at the realization that her eating disorder was no longer working with the same fortitude it had in the past. She had tried to "swallow" her anger toward us, but realized she had still built herself up to be angry enough to contemplate suicide. What she failed to realize at the time was that by expressing her anger she chose a fork: the fork that deals with the reality of her life. That feelings are OK and it's OK to express them. She began to understand that we weren't leaving. If anything, our goal was to encourage her expression of feelings. As she became more comfortable, she began to explain her resistance to sharing her anger with people in the past: there were no underlying guarantees that anything would *change* if she told someone how she felt.

She recalled one of the more clear examples; her mother approached her after an argument with Kaylee's father. Her mother expressed her feelings of anger and confusion regarding her relationship with her husband. She explained to Kaylee how unhappy she was and that she wished she could find a way to get out of her marriage. Kaylee, being the caretaker, allowed her mother to share her feelings, get upset, and ask for suggestions and advice. Kaylee recalled feeling angry toward her mother for not standing up for herself, and angry toward her father for creating so much turmoil. This felt like the thousandth time her mother had come to her, crying the blue about her unhappy marriage, asking Kaylee for advice, and returning to the same pattern each time, never changing anything. Kaylee would struggle with sharing her angry feelings, telling her mother she wished that she and her father would separate, and how much nicer it would be if they weren't arguing all the time.

Kaylee began to recognize two strong perspectives on this situation. One, no matter what she said, suggested, or advised, nothing was going to change; and two, the more things remained the same, the more she began to question her own abilities as a good caretaker. Looking back now, she began to experience the anger she felt at the time in what she describes as a "no-win situation." She couldn't get her own childhood needs met because she was too busy being the caretaker; and she couldn't get her caretaking needs met because every time she switched roles and became the parent, her mother disregarded her suggestions and advice. While remembering and sharing these feelings, Kaylee recognized for the first time that she always felt as though she failed at both parenting and at being a child. Both of these messages epitomize shame-based feelings.

As we sat and talked about this, it became clear that Kaylee was experiencing these feelings of anger and failure with the same intensity as she had when she was a child. And so another fork—one road represents the continuation of those feelings of anger and entrapment, which will follow if a patient chooses to continue to "swallow" them; the other road representing the path to reality, which begins for the patient when she chooses to recognize, acknowledge and express her feelings.

Kaylee spoke with us about this at great length. She stated at the end of the conversation that she was experiencing a tremendous sense of belief. With a somewhat surprised look, she smiled and said the feelings of relief were very similar to the relief she experienced following a purge. She did admit that talking about her feelings was a whole lot harder than "stuffing" them down and flushing them away. Hopefully, each time a patient risks exploring reality, there will be an increase in confidence and self-esteem.

Throughout therapy the eating-disordered person will encounter many forks in the road. When a person becomes "stuck" at a fork, we often ask them "What are you feeding yourself?" More often than not the person looks puzzled and says, "I'm in the middle of telling you what I've been struggling with and you're asking me what I ate today?" We remind her, "You are what you eat." Confused, she struggles with what it is that we're actually asking. (As we mentioned earlier, we would love to re-name this disorder a "feeding disorder." We explain to people that if they become stuck in these areas, it is because that they're feeding themselves negative destructful messages about themselves. If someone fills herself up, or binges on negative messages she becomes negative in her thinking; thus she does become what she eats.)

Although the eating-disordered person is faced with many forks in the road, our experience has been that there are four major crossroads she will encounter. Forks dealing with eating, relationships, family, and self, in that order. The eating behavior most often is a precipitating factor. The person comes into therapy when the eating is out of control. This is the first major fork they are willing to explore. It appears that this is the most threatening issue the person is experiencing, but in reality it is the least threatening of the four major forks. The need to hold onto the eating disorder is a measure of just how threatening the remaining forks are. Interestingly enough, the eating-disordered person starts with the fork in the road that essentially has to do solely with herself. Once the eating behavior becomes more comfortable for her to look at, she moves on to explore interpersonal and intimate relationships, then on again to family issues. Both of these forks involve other people. Finally, the eating-disordered person moves on to the most threatening fork—that of exploring self. This final crossroad in recovery has again to do solely with herself. As the eating-disordered person struggles with these forks in her road, more and more self-confidence begins to build. Choosing the healthier paths counteracts negative messages.

People with eating disorders often say they feel they are the only ones expriencing these struggles, or forks in the road. The reality is that no one escapes having to make choices throughout their lives—some tougher than others. What we do know is that when a person chooses a fork or path to follow, another one is waiting somewhere down the road. That's life.

# 8

# Recovery:
# Follow the Yellow Brick Road

**B**efore Dave and I started working together on the Eating Disorders Program, I had three female inpatients that I was treating. One morning when I arrived at work, I was approached by these three ladies who were excitedly telling me about a story they wanted to share with me. When I told them to meet me in my office in fifteen minutes, they quickly went off, explaining they needed to rehearse it one more time. They also let me know that they thought I would love it. Fifteen minutes later I had three very excited, giggly females in my office. They explained to me that they had all gotten together on the unit the night before, and had begun sharing with each other their true feelings about having an eating disorder. They went on to explain the most wonderful story I've heard—a story that has been repeated many times over, to all my other patients since then. It was the story of the Wizard of Oz. The three patients each felt as though they had all the characteristics of Dorothy, the Tin Man, the Scarecrow, and the Cowardly Lion. They saw Dorothy as the "worrier." She was always worried about Aunty Em and her family. Worrying was a trait all three of these patients were very familiar with. They felt as though they were selfish and heartless like the Tin Man, who felt as though no one could love him, since he did not have a heart that would allow him to love back. They saw themselves as unintelligent like the Scarecrow, who did not have a brain; and because they continually felt afraid of what life had to offer they saw themselves as the Cowardly Lion saw himself. When they put all these characteristics together they felt as though they were looking at themselves. They went on to explain that they felt they were on the yellow brick road looking for recovery. What they found along the way was the Wicked Witch, better known to them as the "bulimic." Just as the Wicked Witch tried to undermine Dorothy's journey back home, they felt that the bulimic tried to undermine their recovery. When things seemed as though they were going OK, the Wicked Witch led Dorothy and her friends into the poppy field, hoping they would fall asleep and never reach the Emerald City. The bulimic, they explained, leads them into the field of depression where they experience a sense of hopelessness that their eating disorder will never end. To my surprise, they saw me as the Good Witch who never really told them what to do, but shared with them some words of wisdom and asked them to never lose faith in themselves. As they continued to battle the wicked bulmic they realized how difficult and long the journey really was going to be. They continued their story, explaining a very significant piece. They asked me if I remembered when Dorothy arrived in the Emerald City, hoping to speak to the Wizard. What they related to was the image of a man as large as a wall, who came across as powerful and controlling . . . until Toto went over and pulled the curtain back, revealing a small man using all his energy to manipulate the control switches to keep that image of the powerful, controlling figure going. Does this seem familiar? As we've mentioned throughout this book, the eating-disordered person spends an incredible amount of energy and time trying to project a powerful, controlling image, when the reality is that inside they are like this little man scrambling to keep the image going.

Finally, these ladies asked me what I thought. I remember not so much what I thought, as what I felt. I felt a sense of happiness that these ladies were able, for their own recovery, to relate to such a classic, well-loved movie. They quickly let me know that there was a moral to this story—and this seemed to be the part that they were most proud of. The moral of the story is that Dorothy always had the power to get home—she just didn't know it.

The same holds true in recovery. Everyone has the power to change, grow, and let go of those issues interfering with their lives.

Many people have asked David and me how recovery happens. Is it when the bingeing and purging stops, or when you are able to feel? Recovery is a process, and a succession of in-roads, relapses, and feelings of success when the *person* is in control *instead* of the eating disorder.

In the last chapter we took a look at the four major forks: eating, relationships, family, and self. When dealing with recovery, it comes to our attention that a fifth fork needs to be added: the fork representing grieving. As the eating-disordered person begins to unravel and understand these different forks, there is a significant amount of grieving going on. Someone once asked us which is more painful—the bulimia or the recovery process. We're not sure how to answer that. With each fork and each decision, there is a process of letting go. When any of us lets go of something that has had any hint of value in our lives we experience a sense of loss.

If we look at the recovery process in terms of the four identified forks we need to start with the eating. Recovery from the eating part of this disorder is—possible. It is important to remember that although it is named an eating disorder, the eating is only a small component of the whole.

It is not uncommon for us to hear that the eating behavior, whether it be restricting, bingeing, and/or purging, increases at the onset of therapy. Many times we have had people start the second or third session by saying that when they left the initial session they experienced a sense of relief and felt some sense of hope. They also add that, unfortunately their eating disorder has become more pronounced. We often tell people at the end of the first sessions to put the "yellow caution light" on. Our experience has been that when a person enters therapy, some part of her (the voice, if you will) becomes threatened and, like so many other times, sees this as a golden opportunity to sabotage recovery. So it is important to know that this is a normal part of the recovery process. The reverse flip side to this is when the person comes into the second or third session reporting that everything is wonderful, and there have been no outward signs of disturbance with her eating. Again, another golden opportunity to sabotage recovery. The end result seems to be the same, whether there is an increase in eating, or a period of time when things are going well. The patients self-confidence and self-esteem both plummet.

It's hard to say which is the most difficult part of recovery from the eating behavior: the beginning, the middle, or the letting go. The beginning seems almost impossible sometimes. For most, bingeing, purging or restricting has been a major obsession that has consumed their thoughts for years. It also feels like a twenty-four-hour-a-day job. The most common statement we hear at the beginning is that the patient has "screwed up" six out of the last seven days. (This is probably a person who has binged, and/or purged, or eaten nothing on a daily basis for the last two or three years.) When we asked about the one good day she almost looks surprised, as if that day doesn't really count in view of the six others that presented difficulty. Taking the eating-disordered person's black-and-white thinking into account, it makes sense that she disregards that one day. It either has to be seven perfect days, or it doesn't count.

At the beginning of recovery, many people ask us to put them on a meal plan, feeling that if they could follow some regimen or know the right foods to eat, they would do better. We try not to get lost in this de-focusing technique! People with eating disorders could publish best-selling books on nutrition and healthy weight loss. Remember, this is their passion. So, it's important not to get too caught up in what's being eaten or what's being done with it. The only time it does become an issue is when there are possible health risks involved. These need to be addressed immediately.

Dealing with the actual eating behavior is probably the most frightening step in the process. The new behavior is based on trial and error. There are no set standards as how to re-incorporate eating into the day, or how to lessen the bingeing and/or purging. One fact we do know is that unlike the alcoholic who, in treatment, learns "don't go to bars or hang out with your drinking and drugging friends," the eating-disordered person must learn throughout recovery to re-incorporate food into her day with some sense of normalcy. The hard part is that the substance we need to survive has become the "enemy." Most people we have treated can recall a period of time before their eating disorder when they felt as though they had normal eating habits. It's important for the patient to remember that she wasn't born with an eating disorder. It entered into her life at a point where feelings were so painful that it seemed easier to self-destruct than to deal with these feelings.

When a person with an eating disorder begins to play with the idea of changing this behavior, it becomes overwhelming. For years, she has accepted this as a part of herself, a part of her daily existence. For years it's gone seemingly unquestioned. Now, there is a recognition that the behavior is abnormal and hurtful to herself.

Guilt is a primary focus we hear from the onset of therapy. Most patients realize the eating part of the disorder is destructive, and more than likely has affected other people; and so starts the guilt.

Another major difficulty is experienced when other people become aware of the person's eating disorder. When a recovering alcoholic at a party refuses a drink from even an insistent host by saying, "No thanks, I don't drink—I'm an alcoholic," everyone understands and there is no pressure and no question. But change the substance offered to food, and the person with an eating disorder gets a very different response. People understand alcoholism—the alcoholic can't drink any more. Most people have a tremendous curiosity about eating disorders because they are not clearly understood.

A problem that makes the eating seem even more difficult is that the eyes of all those who know are on the patient. With the anorexic, putting food into her mouth becomes a major event for those close to her. There is also an expectation of thinness. "If I let these people see me eat, they will expect me to gain weight and then they might think that this is just a phase." It often feels like a no-win situation. In order to start the process of recovery she has to eat; if she eats, she's lost control. For the bulimic or compulsive overeater all eyes also are on what she puts in her mouth. For the bulimic, there is an extra stress because everyone panics when she heads for the bathroom after a meal. What's difficult to accept is that the eating part of the disorder has violated others' trust. The anorexic is manipulative, stating she ate three meals that day when the reality could be that she ate three carrot sticks. The bulimic swears she hasn't purged, yet there are traces of it in the bathroom. The compulsive eater swears she stuck to her meal plan—at the same time she's trying to find hiding places for the empty wrappers; and so trust becomes violated. This is one of the most annoying parts for the eating-disordered person who is trying her best to get the eating under control. I can remember vividly the tension surrounding meals during the beginning of my recovery process. When I finally stopped purging I felt as though I had really hit a milestone. I was still overeating, but to be rid of the purging felt nothing short of heaven. I have always had a tendency to drink soda or iced tea with a meal. Understandably, I would have to relieve myself shortly thereafter. What I taught my family when I was actively purging was "I'm on my way to the bathroom to get rid of the food." When I wasn't doing this any more, it became increasingly frustrating every time I was questioned as to what I was doing in the bathroom. Many times at the beginning of this new-found freedom from purging, my mother would knock on the bathroom door asking what I was doing, and when I responded that I was just going to the bathroom, she would hesitate and wait until I came out. Finally, after feeling the mistrust, I would invite her into the bathroom, if this was what she felt she needed to do to verify what was happening. Most often she would sit in the bathroom while I relieved myself, talking about the day's events. This lasted for quite a long time until I think she finally realized I was doing OK. It provoked a tremendous amount of guilt and anger. I felt guilty that I had created such turmoil and angry that now, when I was serious about recovery, no one was trusting my efforts. I can also recall saying many times that recovery is not worth it—nobody believes me anyway. What we do know about people who fall into eating disorders is that they have an incredible amount of strength within. Unfortunately, this strength somehow gets channeled into a destructive mode. Recovery from an eating disorder requires all of this strength. It's important to keep going even when it seems like it's hopeless.

As the eating behavior decreases (and it can), the eating-disordered person most often experiences tremendous mood swings. Not only does the bingeing and/or purging take on a less than acceptable value, but the same feelings that created the eating disorder still surface. Many parents or significant others report that the mood swings are sometimes unbearable. What the outsider has not been able to experience is the internal struggle the eating-disordered person has been dealing with. It becomes increasingly evident when an outsider watches the person go from incredible highs to devastating lows. This middle step, as we refer to it, is the most painful emotionally. The eating-disordered person begins to let go of the eating behavior and begins to panic about what life is really about. One of the most difficult tasks is to sit through the feelings of wanting to binge; or, following a binge, to sit through the feelings of wanting to purge. We feel it's important when talking about this stage of recovery to address the issue of weight gain. Very often, when the purging ceases but the bingeing continues, the patient will experience a weight gain. The weight gain can vary from a few pounds to many pounds. (One of the experiences I shared in the introduction came after seven months of intensive therapy, when my therapist recommended a diet.) Unfortunately, what this weight gain does is increase the chances for a binge. Throughout recovery, the eating-disordered person will find herself still obsessed with her weight, even to the point of wanting to go back to dieting. Remember, these thoughts are normal but she has to put the yellow caution light on when thinking of actually acting on these feelings.

The recovering patient will find herself experiencing a tremendous amount of frustration. Trial and error is not the easiest concept to deal with—mainly because trial and error takes patience and determination. Determination, the eating-disordered person has. Patience—well that's something else. During this middle phase, *everything* seems exaggerated. We had a patient in the hospital recently who went on one of our famous grocery shopping adventures mentioned earlier. What she reported after leaving the store was that she felt as though everything was louder; the noise, the people, even the colors on the food wrappers. It's important to remember that awareness is increasing, while at the same time her head is clearing of many obsessive thoughts.

The eating-disordered person finds herself returning to

old behaviors in situations where she's not feeling strong enough to reach out for better coping mechanisms. What we do know is that throughout the steps of recovery she will experience a return to old behaviors at least a few times, if not more. That's normal, and part of the process. Remember, it's not the end of the world (although it can sure feel like that sometimes). Throughout this process food becomes more and more integrated into the patient's life. The key to this process is how she feels about herself. Food will always be there to hide behind. She has to be the one to decide to come out of hiding.

Fully letting go of the control eating has had over her life takes time, a lot of time. It's a normal and common part of the process to continue to have the thoughts of wanting to restrict, binge and/or purge. The patient has to step back when these feelings overtake her and ask herself "What am I really trying to communicate through my bingeing or restricting?" Also, it's important for her to understand that the bingeing may come upon her at a time when things seem as though they're going relatively well. She may not always be able to pinpoint or understand a reason for her bingeing. But people with eating disorders are wonderful during a crisis or times of undue stress. It's the delayed reaction (which can be a matter of a few hours or a few weeks) that creates uncomfortable feelings.

We've taken a look at the first fork of eating. Throughout the remaining forks it's important to remember the eating disorder may still be active to some degree. We do not want to present the eating as something that must be under control before the other forks are addressed.

The second fork in the recovery process deals with the issue of relationships. Throughout recovery an integral part is the awareness of the relationships the eating-disordered person has experienced throughout her life. The most common and painful issue we hear regarding relationships is the feeling of not belonging. Most people we've encountered state that they always felt as though they were on the periphery of a group. This feeling is one of never fitting in as well as those who appear to be the center of the group. What makes looking at relationships a complex part of recovery is that the eating-disordered person almost always sees it only one way—"it must be something about *me* that people dislike." It's hard for her to recognize that a relationship always consists of more than one person. Recovery involves taking a very honest look at relationships. The patient will usually find that the relationships she has established involved either caretaking or control. When it was caretaking, it was easy to not allow the other to really know her, since the main focus was on taking care of that other. When it was trying to maintain control or have the upper hand, she allowed other people in only as far as she wanted them. Both represent lopsided relationships.

Isolation has also played a major role during the eating disorder, and therefore, most relationships have suffered in some way. Throughout recovery it is important to re-evaluate past and present relationships. The most significant is the relationship with self, which is something we will be taking a look at later on in this chapter. What we do know is that until a sound relationship with self develops it remains difficult to make amends with others. So much time has been spent by the eating-disordered person beating herself up that little room is left to put damaged relationships back together. I can clearly recall coming home from college at eighty-six pounds and seeing the fellow I had dated throughout high school. His response was most likely one of fear. He told me he couldn't stand to look at me this way—much less continue to see me. At the time I was so consumed with my disorder that those words seemed almost insignificant. It wasn't until a year and a half later, when my feet were more firmly on the ground and my head more clear, that we were able to talk about what had happened. I'm glad we were able to re-establish a friendship. My dearest friends (better known as the M. G. 7's, to whom this book is dedicated) never really left my side. I'm not sure if they understood what I had done to myself, or why, but they never left me. There were times when they would call and ask me if I wanted to go to Friendly's with them. I could remember saying to myself "What—are these guys nuts? They know I can't go to Friendly's for an ice cream." What they were really doing was including me in things. In fact there were times I'd go to Friendly's with them and have a diet soda while they enjoyed their ice cream. The key factor was the company.

On the other hand there were relationships that were so damaged that they were irreparable. Here again, there is a tremendous sense of guilt. Until the feelings of guilt become more clearly understood within the self it's difficult to express these feelings to others.

Hopefully throughout recovery the patient will learn and understand the destruction of addiction. When reevaluating the relationships it's important to be honest enough with herself to look at those relationships that have an addictive nature. One thing to be careful of is to not transfer her obsession with eating or weight to another obsession or addiction. Once she allows herself to spend less time obsessing on issues she is able to spend more time developing and cultivating healthy relationships.

Everyone wants both to feel needed and to have a sense of fitting in. The important insight is that it has to come from within.

The third fork deals with family. Of the two forks that deal with other people, family is the most difficult. Without mincing words, the family system has a major role in the eating disorder. Most people with eating disorders feel as though they don't fit into the family unit. Sometimes this is realistic and sometimes it's not. This is not to say the family is to blame. What we are suggesting is that the combination of the messages given to a young child and how this child perceives them is an important part of the foundation of an eating disorder. It's difficult for any of us to experience a family member in either emotional or physical pain—especially when this pain is self-imposed. Throughout recovery it becomes vital to take stock in relationships with family. Most often it is centered around parents and siblings. When working on this issue we often ask that the eating-disordered person begin to see her parents as people. They will always be mom and dad, but just as she is taking a step back to look at herself and the person she presents to the world, it's equally important to view her parents in the same way. What type of people are they and what traits do they bring into their own relationships? Unfortunately, she may not always like the people she sees. In the past, this was never questioned, but because recovery means questioning everything, it cannot be untouched.

The eating disorder itself has more than likely disrupted the family system. Even though it feels like the patient is the only person going through it, the family members in some way go through it with her. This in itself presents another fork. She can spend much of her time, energy, and effort feeling badly or guilty for having put them through this whole ordeal *or* she can accept that it has happened and continue on the yellow brick road. We're not saying it's as easy as it sounds, just a little "food for thought," as they say.

Our experience has been that dealing with family issues in and of itself creates a tremendous amount of upheaval. What the person with an eating disorder likes to disregard sometimes is that although family is family, they cannot read minds. The family only knows what she shares with them. Remember, in dysfunctional families a key component that is usually missing is the ability to communicate how one feels.

During recovery the eating-disordered person almost always experiences a sense of frustration when dealing with the family and the surrounding issues. A family system is like a mobile. When one part is taken out all the other parts are affected. Another way to look at this: when a rusty part is taken out of something, fixed, cleaned up and put back, it is being put back in with other rusty parts that haven't been cleaned up. So when the person in recovery looks at family issues, understands and begins to confront them, frustration builds because the rest of the family may not have taken a look or changed their perspective on things. This is one of the most common complaints we hear. And yet more forks: stay in the family dwelling or leave, accepting that things aren't going to change; suggest family therapy or (what one experienced in the past) go back to the old behaviors because it's less painful—or seems so—than fighting the odds. Remember recovery is a process. The patient may find herself doing all of the above at one time or another. The most important part is to take care of herself. This may sound selfish and maybe it is, but it's self against self in the end—which brings us to the fourth fork: self. Throughout the entire book we have been mentioning self in one form or another. Another word for recovery is liking oneself. That's what recovery is truly all about. How does one do that? By allowing herself to look at all the hard and painful issues in her life and by nurturing all the good that's already there. Throughout the recovery process it's important to address the child within. Many people begin to cry when we ask them about this child. Why? Because they know she's in there hiding from all of the hurt and pain. Looking at self is looking at this child. This is the one who, for whatever reason, was kept trapped inside the body. This is the fun part, the silly side of each of us. The one who would love nothing more than to be spontaneous; spontaneous with eating, relationships, family, life in general. Our understanding is that it is very difficult to be spontaneous and in control at the same time. Recovery means letting go of a lot of control. That doesn't mean giving other people control, it simply means maybe there isn't any real need to control situations. What appears to happen is that control comes to take up too much time—there are always questions like, "Should I laugh at the person's joke? What happens if I pick a movie for everyone to see and it's a bomb—will they all dislike me because I made a bad choice?"

When re-evaluating self, humor plays an integral role. Everything feels so serious all the time. How could it not when a person has to go through the third degree every time she makes a decision. Accepting self means to be able to laugh at the things she's done and realize she's human. It means breaking away from that black-and-white thinking where everything is either good or bad, right or wrong. Maybe there are more than just two ways of looking at everything. Accepting self means taking care of oneself *before* taking care of others, rather than taking care of others *instead* of taking care of oneself. That statement is saying "Yeah, you're a caretaker and that's a nice quality to have, but make sure you're doing OK first." We look at the issues with control, caretaking and perfectionism as always being a part of each patient. It's like a stereo system. There are knobs which control the degree of balance, loudness, forward, reverse and pause. It's the same with self. Each person can regulate the degree to which these issues affect her life. Taking a step back can help her realize these qualities could be good healthy ones as long as she channels the energy into a positive, constructive direction.

Just like the child within who's been in hiding, all the other qualities that will be brought out and nurtured throughout therapy have also been in hiding. We let people know that they probably won't learn anything drastically new about themselves. It's all in there. It's just being pushed down by a tremendous amount of fear. Recovery is the removal, almost block by block, of that fear, until it feels safe to bring that little child out. For some, this recovery process takes a few years; others battle it for a lifetime. Is it possible to recover? Yes. This is not to say, though, that life will stop presenting all of us with some difficult forks along the way. What the patient will gain throughout recovery is the sense of strength and confidence she needs to confront these forks and move on.

When discussing this chapter on recovery we felt a need to include a fork dealing with the grieving process. As we've seen throughout the book, recovery signifies letting go and moving ahead. Along with this, there is grieving over those losses. The grieving process is similar in many respects to the process surrounding death and dying. Elisabeth Kübler-Ross wrote in her book *On Death and Dying* (New York: Macmillan, 1969) about the five stages: denial, anger, depression, bargaining and acceptance. We would like to end the book by looking at how these five stages need to be addressed with the eating-disordered person throughout recovery.

Initially with most eating-disordered people there is denial. Denial within themselves, and denial to the rest of the world that there is anything wrong. Like the person who finds out they are dying and denies this could be happening to them, the eating-disordered person also denies they have a problem and that their behavior is abnormal. This stage can last for as long as the person wishes it to. As painful as it is to acknowledge, we believe that underneath that fear the eating-disordered person realizes what they really are doing. When the need to deny is no longer as prevalent, a second stage becomes evident. When terminally ill people understand they're dying, they become filled with anger that this is happening to them. "Why me? What did I do to deserve this?" They feel as though life has played a trick on them. They feel cheated. The eating-disordered person feels very similar, asking similar questions. "Why am I the kid in the family who gets this thing? How come everybody else can deal with issues and I can't?" This anger needs to be addressed and processed out. Most often during this anger stage, depression begins to creep in. There is a sudden realization that no matter how angry the person gets it's still a very real situation. The stages of anger and depression seem to overlap throughout the course of recovery. Then comes the bargaining. Terminally ill people begin to make all sorts of amends. If they're allowed to get better they'll go to church every Sunday, they'll never say another bad thing about anybody. The eating-disordered person also begins to bargain. She'll give up the eating disorder and all the trimmings if someone will guarantee her that she won't gain weight or that she'll always be accepted and loved. Finally terminally ill people begin to accept that this is real and it's life's plan for them. They become more at peace with themselves, and most often reassure those around them that this is really OK. The major difference during this final acceptance stage for the eating-disordered person is that she does have a choice. She doesn't need to accept that she is going to die. She needs to accept herself for who she is. She needs to love, nurture and support herself in whatever endeavors she faces. Accepting herself is giving herself another chance at life—one that does not have to be so confusing or painful.

The eating-disordered person grieves for many things throughout the recovery process. Initially there is the loss of hiding behind a substance—food—to deal with life. There is a loss of some significant relationships. There is a loss felt from giving up whatever role she played in the family, and separating emotionally from those family members; and finally there is the loss of therapy and the therapist. All of these losses need to be addressed, for without fully grieving there remains a feeling of unfinished business.

With each loss there is a gain. Life without an eating disorder allows the person time to explore and to take from it what she may. New relationships are formed and the old ones are reintroduced. Separating and letting go is a healthy, normal part of life. One thing we both cherish is hearing from people who we've dealt within the past, calling us to "just say hello." There comes a clear understanding that the needs they once had in any relationship have changed. They don't need people the same way anymore. It's just nice to know that they're there.

We hope that you've enjoyed the book. One thing we know is that it was written from our hearts. We would like to leave you with a poem one of our patients wrote upon terminating therapy. It's called *Witch Traps,* after the infamous wicked witch of bulimia and remember, "Dorothy always had the power to get home—She just didn't know it." So do all eating-disordered people.

## Witch Traps

When I first started across the woods
I wanted you to show me
Where all the witch traps were,
If not be there every time I stumbled on to one.
But, you would only describe what they looked like,
and forged on ahead telling me to think about
exactly how I might handle the witches
should I chance to run into one.
I must admit now
that I did see you peek out from behind the trees
in the near distance
every once in awhile,
and whisper piercingly, so that I had to hear,
"Remember to check the vegetation
and use your judgment."
And I chanced upon a lot of traps in the darkness,
and got chased and cursed and hexed
and all of the other things sneaky witches will do
more than a few times,
although not by anything too evil.
And between commercials
I managed to start to decipher a path
strewn conveniently with a few friends,
and slowly get used to the technicolor

that was a far cry from the Kansas black and white.
Now I have learned enough to consider writing a book,
entitled, "The Fine Art of Placating Witches."
And I've gotten so good lately,
that next week I've decided
to start working on Warlock holes
before heading home.

# Appendix A

The Twelve Steps of Recovery Adapted from Alcoholics Anonymous*

1. We admitted we were powerless over food—that our lives had become unmanageable.

2. Came to believe that a Power greater than ourselves could restore us to sanity.

3. Made a decision to turn our will and our lives over to the care of God *as we understood Him.*

4. Made a searching and fearless moral inventory of ourselves.

5. Admitted to God, to ourselves, and to another human being, the exact nature of our wrongs.

6. Were entirely ready to have God remove all these defects of character.

7. Humbly asked Him to remove our shortcomings.

8. Made a list of all persons we had harmed, and became willing to make amends to them all.

9. Made direct amends to such people wherever possible, except when to do so would injure them or others.

10. Continued to take personal inventory and when we were wrong promptly admitted it.

11. Sought through prayer and meditation to improve our conscious contact with God *as we understood Him,* praying only for knowledge of His will for us and the power to carry that out.

12. Having had a spiritual awakening as the result of these steps, we tried to carry this message to compulsive overeaters, and to practice these principles in all our affairs.

*The Twelve Steps are reprinted with permission of Alcoholics Anonymous World Services, Inc. Permission to reprint and adapt the Twelve Steps does not mean that A.A. is in any way affiliated with this program. A.A. is a program of recovery from alcoholism. Use of the Twelve Steps in connection with programs and activities which are patterned after A.A. but which address other problems does not imply otherwise.

## The Twelve Steps of Alcoholics Anonymous

1. We admitted we were powerless over alcohol—that our lives had become unmanageable. 2. Came to believe that a Power greater than ourselves could restore us to sanity. 3. Made a decision to turn our will and our lives over to the care of God *as we understood Him.* 4. Made a searching and fearless moral inventory of ourselves. 5. Admitted to God, to ourselves, and to another human being the exact nature of our wrongs. 6. Were entirely ready to have God remove all these defects of character. 7. Humbly asked Him to remove our shortcomings. 8. Made a list of all persons we had harmed, and became willing to make amends to them all. 9. Made direct amends to such people wherever possible, except when to do so would injure them or others. 10. Continued to take personal inventory and when we were wrong promptly admitted it. 11. Sought through prayer and meditation to improve our conscious contact with God, *as we understood Him,* praying only for knowledge of His will for us and the power to carry that out. 12. Having had a spiritual awakening as the result of these steps, we tried to carry this message to alcoholics, and to practice these principles in all our affairs.

# Introduction to
# Appendices B, C, and D

We felt it was important to include the following information for our readers—therapists, families, and those experiencing the eating disorder—to help everyone better understand the workings of an inpatient program. Placing a loved one in an inpatient program can be a trying but important decision to make.

# Appendix B

The following is a behavioral contract appropriate for Nancy during her fourth week of hospitalization. At that time she was confined to the unit because of unacceptable behavior during the previous week. This behavior included one episode of minor self-injury (scratching herself with a plastic fork), two incidents of eating unauthorized food, and a hostile verbal outburst toward a member of the nursing staff during which she tipped over a chair. At this point in her treatment she had no off-unit privileges except two hours each evening in the recreation room with close supervision by nursing staff.

## Behavioral Contract

Name: Nancy
Date: 10/10/86
Week of hospitalization: 4th

I. Eating
   A. Goal Behaviors
      1. Patient will eat all food on her tray at all meals.
      2. Patient will not eat any food other than in #1.
      3. Patient will meet twice weekly with the dietician to plan meals.
      4. Patient will not vomit or engage in unauthorized physical exercise.

B. Consequences
   1. If the patient accomplishes 1-4 through 10/17/86 bathroom will be left unlocked after meals and 1 to 1 nursing observation during meals will be discontinued.
   2. Failure to accomplish 1-4 will result in bathroom remaining locked for two hours after meals and continued 1 to 1 nursing observation during meals.
   3. If patient is found exercising in her room, further restrictions (1 to 1 in room; lock out of room except between 11 p.m. and 7 a.m.; loss of recreation room privilege) may be imposed at the discretion of the program coordinator.

II. Self-injury
   A. Goal Behaviors
      1. Patient will not cause injury to herself by cutting, scratching, bruising herself, etc.
      2. Patient will express feelings and self-destructive impulses verbally to a member of the treatment team or to co-patients during group therapy.
      3. Patient may use punching dummy with supervision at discretion of nursing staff.
   B. Consequences
      1. If patient accomplishes 1-3 through 10/17/86 she will be allowed to go on bowling and movie trips.
      2. Self-injury will result in confinement to the unit for a minimum of seven days.
      3. Additional restrictions and/or loss of privileges may be imposed at the discretion of the program coordinator.

III. Aggressive Behavior
   A. Goal Behaviors
      1. Patient will express anger verbally in assertive, non-blameful and non-threatening ways.

2. Patient will not physicallly or verbally abuse or threaten any other person.

   a. Any member of the hospital staff is authorized to determine whether a particular behavior is abusive or threatening.

3. Patient will not physically act out anger toward inanimate objects (e.g. throwing, kicking, punching, slamming doors, etc.).

4. Patient may use punching dummy with supervision at the discretion of the nursing staff.

B. Consequences

1. Same as per II.

2. Same as per II.

It will be noted that the contract allows the program coordinator some latitude in imposing consequences for unacceptable behavior. No attempt is made to spell out all consequences in detail. We have found that somewhat "loose" contracts like this one work best because they are more in step with the way the outside world actually is, and because it is impossible to foresee and write down all possible behaviors and extenuating circumstances. Generally, behavioral contracts of this type are reviewed and revised on a weekly basis. The procedure we use for negotiating behavioral contracts with our patients is described in chapter 5.

# Appendix C

## Information For New Patients

### *Admission:*

Initially you will be admitted to the hospital's closed unit. Your length of stay on the closed unit could vary from a few days to several weeks depending on your condition and your ability to function independently.

On the closed unit you will be closely supervised by nursing staff. You will be allowed off the unit for scheduled therapies, but your activities will be closely monitored. Later, when you move to the open unit, you will have more freedom to come and go without supervision.

Certain items are not allowed in patient's rooms on the closed unit (razors, sharp objects, glass containers, etc.). At the time of admission, a nurse will explain the unit rules and go through your belongings with you. Items not allowed in patient rooms are kept in the nursing station and will be available for your use with nursing supervision.

### *Initial Evaluation*

The initial evaluation includes physical examination by an internist, a battery of blood tests and urinalysis, an electrocardiogram, and an electroencephalogram. Psychological testing is also obtained on all patients soon after admission. These evaluations provide a thorough screening for physical problems and baseline information which will help us to plan your treatment and evaluate your progress. If physical problems are present, consultants are available for specialîzed evaluation and treatment when needed.

### *Program Outline:*

You will be scheduled to participate in most or all of the various aspects of the Eating Disorders Program soon after your admission. Each week you will be scheduled for several group therapy sessions, appointments with various members of the Eating Disorders Team, recreational activities, arts and crafts, art therapy, dance therapy, and physical exercise. You will also be seen by the dietitian from time to time to discuss meal planning and nutrition.

In art therapy, dance therapy, and most of your group therapy sessions, you will be with other patients who have eating disorders. We have designed the program in this way because most patients find that having group activities just for eating-disordered patients helps them to focus on important issues and provides a supportive environment for self-understanding and problem solving. In other activities (recreation, physical exercise, arts and crafts) patients with other types of problems will also be present.

### *Eating Related Issues:*

Since you are coming here largely because of problems related to eating, such things as diet, exercise and access to food, bathrooms, laxatives, and diuretics may necessarily be important issues in your treatment and ultimate recovery. Initially, the treatment team will assume control over these aspects of your life insofar as they are of significance in your illness. Meals will be prescribed much as drugs are prescribed for other conditions. Access to bathrooms may be restricted during certain times or allowed only with nursing supervision. Laxatives, diuretics, and other drugs are rarely used in the program and then only when prescribed by your attending psychiatrist. For certain patients, physical exercise may be either restricted or prescribed.

As your treatment progresses, control over these aspects of your life will gradually be turned over to you. The rate at which this will occur is different for each patient and will depend on numerous factors which will be discussed with you during the course of your treatment.

### *Privileges:*

As your condition improves, you will be allowed various privileges. These may include such things as permission to have visitors; to participate in various recreational activities; to walk on hospital grounds without staff supervision; to participate in off-grounds activities; to eat in the central dining room; or to move to the open unit. During the course of your hospital stay, the treatment team may also decide to suspend or revoke one or more privileges. This will only be done for therapeutic reasons and, if this does occur, the reasons will be explained to you.

Decisions about privileges are made by the Program Coordinator with input from other members of the treatment team. Requests for privileges should be made to the Program Coordinator.

### *Passes:*

Except in unusual circumstances, passes are not allowed during the initial evaluation period. Thereafter, as your condition improves, you may be allowed to leave the hospital to attend to personal business or to spend time with family or friends. In determining passes, the following guidelines apply:

1. Passes are for specified periods of time and require the approval of the Eating Disorders Program staff.
2. Passes will be granted for identified therapeutic purposes. For example, testing your ability to control

eating behavior outside the structure of the hospital, or to deal with a conflict in your relationship with a family member, etc.

3. In case of an emergency or special circumstance, a pass may be granted so you can deal with the specific situation.

4. Since you are coming to Craig House for treatment of a serious illness, passes cannot be given for purely "recreational" purposes.

5. During your stay, one overnight pass is allowed. This is usually scheduled near the end of your hospital stay to help you re-adjust to living outside the hospital.

# Appendix D

## Inpatient Daily Schedule

*Monday:*
         9:00 a.m. – Exercise
         9:45 a.m. – Weigh-in
      10:00 a.m. – Individual Therapy
      11:00 a.m. – Group Therapy
      12:00      – Lunch
        1:15 p.m. – Family Issues Group
    *2:30 p.m. – Gym
    *3:30 p.m. – Art Therapy
        5:30 p.m. – Dinner
**7:00–9:00 p.m. – Outside Groups

*Tuesday:*
         9:00 a.m. – Exercise
      10:00 a.m. – Individual Therapy
      11:00 a.m. – Group Therapy
      12:00      – Lunch
        1:15 p.m. – Therapeutic Contracting
        2:30 p.m. – Dance Movement Therapy
    *3:30 p.m. – Arts & Crafts
        5:30 p.m. – Dinner
**7:00–9:00 p.m. – Outside Groups

*Wednesday:*
         9:00 a.m. – Exercise
      10:00 a.m. – Individual Therapy
      11:00 a.m. – Family Issues Group

161

```
                    12:00      − Lunch
                    1:15 p.m. − Grocery Shopping Trip
                   *2:30 p.m. − Gym
                    3:30 p.m. − Art Therapy
                    5:30 p.m. − Dinner
             **7:00−9:00 p.m. − Outside Groups
```

*Thursday:*
```
                    9:00 a.m. − Exercise
                   10:00 a.m. − Individual Therapy
                   11:00 a.m. − Group Therapy
                   12:00      − Lunch
                    1:15 p.m. − Food Lab
                    2:30 p.m. − Dance Movement Therapy
                   *3:30 p.m. − Arts & Crafts
                    5:30 p.m. − Dinner
             **7:00−9:00 p.m. − Outside Groups
```

*Friday:*
```
                    9:00 a.m. − Exercise
                   10:00 a.m. − Individual Therapy
                   11:00 a.m. − Group Therapy
                   12:00      − Lunch
                    1:15 p.m. − Therapeutic Contracting
                                 Group
                   *2:30 p.m. − Gym
                   *3:30 p.m. − Arts & Crafts
                    5:30 p.m. − Dinner
             **7:00−9:00 p.m. − Outside Groups
```

*Often during Gym and Arts & Crafts time patients are seen for individual or family therapy sessions.

**There are outside group meetings such as A.A., O.A., N.A., Al-Anon, and ACoA, that patients may attend. Participation is determined by the eating-disorders team.

# Suggested Reading

Bradshaw, J. 1988. *Healing The Shame That Binds You*. Deerfield Beach, FL: Health Communications, Inc.

Erikson, E. 1968. *Childhood And Society*. New York: Norton.

Kübler-Ross, E. 1969. *On Death And Dying*. New York: Macmillan Publishing, Co.

Levenkron, S. 1979. *The Best Little Girl In the World*. New York: Warner Books.

O'Gorman, P. and Oliver-Diaz, P. 1990. *Self-Parenting 12 Step Workbook*. Deerfield Beach, FL: Health Communications, Inc.

Sandbek, T. 1986. *The Deadly Diet*. Oakland, CA: New Harbinger Publications, Inc.

Siegel, M., Brisman, J., and Weinshel, M. 1988. *Surviving An Eating Disorder: Strategies For Family And Friends*. New York: Harper & Row.

Wholey, D. 1988. New York: Harper & Row, 1988. *Becoming Your Own Parent: The Solution For ACOA And Other Dysfunctional Families*. New York: Bantam Books.

Woititz, J. 1985. *Struggle For Intimacy*. Deerfield Branch, FL: Health Communications, Inc.

# THE CONTINUUM
# COUNSELING LIBRARY
## Books of Related Interest

_____Denyse Beaudet
ENCOUNTERING THE MONSTER
*Pathways in Children's Dreams*
Based on original empirical research, and with recourse to
the works of Jung, Neumann, Eliade, Marie-Louise Franz,
and others, this book offers proven methods of approaching
and understanding the dream life of children. $17.95

_____Robert W. Buckingham
CARE OF THE DYING CHILD
*A Practical Guide for Those Who Help Others*
"Buckingham's book delivers a powerful, poignant message
deserving a wide readership."—*Library Journal* $17.95

_____Alastair V. Campbell, ed.
A DICTIONARY OF PASTORAL CARE
Provides information on the essentials of counseling and the
kinds of problems encountered in pastoral practice. The
approach is interdenominational and interdisciplinary.
Contains over 300 entries by 185 authors in the fields of
theology, philosophy, psychology, and sociology as well as
from the theoretical background of psychotherapy and
counseling. $24.50

_____David A. Crenshaw
BEREAVEMENT
*Counseling the Grieving throughout the Life Cycle*
Grief is examined from a life cycle perspective, infancy to
old age. Special losses and practical strategies for frontline
caregivers highlight this comprehensive guidebook. $16.95

———John Gerdtz and Joel Bregman, M.D.
**AUTISM**
*A Practical Guide for Those Who Help Others*
An up-to-date and comprehensive guidebook for everyone who works with autistic children, adolescents, adults, and their families. Includes latest information on medications. $16.95

———Marion Howard
**HOW TO HELP YOUR TEENAGER**
**POSTPONE SEXUAL INVOLVEMENT**
Based on a national educational program that works, this book advises parents, teachers, and counselors on how they can help their teens resist social and peer pressures regarding sex. $14.95

———Marion Howard
**SOMETIMES I WONDER ABOUT ME**
*Teenagers and Mental Health*
Combines fictional narratives with sound, understandable professional advice to help teenagers recognize the difference between serious problems and normal problems of adjustment. $9.95

———E. Clay Jorgensen
**CHILD ABUSE**
*A Practical Guide for Those Who Help Others*
Essential information and practical advice for caregivers called upon to help both child and parent in child abuse. $16.95

———Eugene Kennedy
**CRISIS COUNSELING**
*The Essential Guide for Nonprofessional Counselors*
"An outstanding author of books on personal growth selects types of personal crises that our present life style has made commonplace and suggests effective ways to deal with them."—*Best Sellers* $11.95

_____Eugene Kennedy and Sara Charles, M.D.
ON BECOMING A COUNSELOR
*A Basic Guide for Nonprofessional Counselors*
New expanded edition of an indispensable resource. A
patient-oriented, clinically directed field guide to
understanding and responding to troubled people. $27.95
hardcover $15.95 paperback

_____Eugene Kennedy
SEXUAL COUNSELING
*A Practical Guide for Those Who Help Others*
Newly revised and up-to-date edition, with a new chapter on
[the counselor and] AIDS, of an essential book on
counseling people with sexual problems. $17.95

_____Bonnie Lester
WOMEN AND AIDS
*A Practical Guide for Those Who Help Others*
Provides positive ways to women to deal with their fears, and
to help others who react with fear to people who have AIDS.
$15.95

_____Robert J. Lovinger
RELIGION AND COUNSELING
*The Psychological Impact of Religious Belief*
How counselors and clergy can best understand the
important emotional significance of religious thoughts and
feelings. $17.95

_____Helen B. McDonald and Audrey I. Steinhorn
HOMOSEXUALITY
*A Practical Guide to Counseling Gays, Lesbians, and Their Families*
A sensitive guide to better understanding and counseling
gays, lesbians, and their parents, at every stage of their lives.
$16.95

_____Paul G. Quinnett
SUICIDE: THE FOREVER DECISION
*For Those Thinking About Suicide,*
*and For Those Who Know, Love, or Counsel Them*
"A treasure—this book can help save lives. It will be
especially valuable not only to those who are thinking about
suicide but to such nonprofessional counselors as teachers,
clergy, doctors, nurses, and to experienced therapists."—
William Van Ornum, psychotherapist and author $18.95
hardcover $8.95 paperback

_____Paul G. Quinnett
THE TROUBLED PEOPLE BOOK
A practical and positive guide to the world of psychotherapy
and psychotherapists. "Without a doubt one of the most
honest, reassuring, nonpaternalistic, and useful self-help
books ever to appear."—*Booklist* $9.95

_____Judah L. Ronch
ALZHEIMER'S DISEASE
*A Practical Guide for Those Who Help Others*
Must reading for everyone—from family members to
professional caregivers—who must deal with the effects of
this tragic disease on a daily basis. Filled with illustrative
examples as well as facts, this book provides sensitive insights
into dealing with one's feelings as well as with such practical
advice as how to choose long-term care. $17.95

_____Theodore Isaac Rubin, M.D.
ANTI-SEMITISM: A DISEASE OF THE MIND
"A most poignant and lucid psychological examination of a
severe emotional disease. Dr. Rubin offers hope and
understanding to the victim and to the bigot. A splendid
job!"—Dr. Herbert S. Strean $14.95

_____John R. Shack
COUPLES COUNSELING
*A Practical Guide for Those Who Help Others*
An essential guide to dealing with the 20 percent of all
counseling situations that involve the relationship of two
people. $15.95

_____Stuart Sutherland
## THE INTERNATIONAL DICTIONARY OF PSYCHOLOGY
This new dictionary of psychology also covers a wide range of related disciplines, from anthropology to sociology. $49.95

_____Joan Leslie Taylor
## IN THE LIGHT OF DYING
*The Journals of a Hospice Volunteer*
A rare and beautiful book about death and dying that affirms life and will inspire an attitude of love. "Beautifully recounts the healing (our own) that results from service to others, and might well be considered as required reading for hospice volunteers."—Stephen Levine $17.95

_____Montague Ullman, M.D. and Claire Limmer, M.S., eds.
## THE VARIETY OF DREAM EXPERIENCE
*Expanding Our Ways of Working With Dreams*
"Lucidly describes the beneficial impact dream analysis can have in diverse fields and in society as a whole. An erudite, illuminating investigation."—*Booklist* $19.95 hardcover $14.95 paperback

_____William Van Ornum and Mary W. Van Ornum
## TALKING TO CHILDREN ABOUT NUCLEAR WAR
"A wise book. A needed book. An urgent book."—Dr. Karl A. Menninger $15.95 hardcover $7.95 paperback

_____Kathleen Zraly and David Swift, M.D.
## ANOREXIA, BULIMIA, AND COMPULSIVE OVEREATING
*A Practical Guide for Counselors and Families*
A psychiatrist and an eating-disorders specialist provide new and helpful approaches for everyone who knows, loves, or counsels victims of anorexia, bulimia, and chronic overeating. $17.95

At your bookstore, or to order directly, send your check or money order (adding $2.00 extra per book for postage and handling, up to $6.00 maximum) to: The Continuum Publishing Company, 370 Lexington Avenue, New York, NY, 10017. Prices are subject to change.